Compliments of
McNeil Laboratories
AND
John Pawlos

CLINICAL

PSYCHOPHARMACOLOGY

Jerrold G. Bernstein, M.D., Editor
Associate Medical Director, Human Resource Institute of Boston; Assistant Clinical Professor of Psychiatry, Harvard Medical School; Assistant Psychiatrist, Massachusetts General Hospital, Boston, Massachusetts

PSG Publishing Company, Inc.
Littleton, Massachusetts

Library of Congress Cataloging in Publication Data
Main entry under title:

Clinical psychopharmacology.

  1. Psychopharmacology. I. Bernstein, Jerrold G.,
1941-   [DNLM: 1. Mental Disorders—Drug therapy.
2. Psychopharmacology. WM402 C641]
RC483.C54   615'.78   76-15733
ISBN 0-88416-176-5

Printed in the United States of America.

International Standard Book Number: 0-88416-176-5

Library of Congress Catalog Card Number: 76-15733

To my wife, Arlene, and our children, Janet and David, and to *Shalom Ba'it*.

Say not anything that cannot be understood, in the hope that it will be understood in the end, and do not say: "When I have leisure I will study"; perchance you may never have leisure.

Hillel, *Pirke Avot*

CONTRIBUTORS

Jerrold G. Bernstein, M.D.
Associate Medical Director
Human Resource Institute of
  Boston
Assistant Clinical Professor of
  Psychiatry
Harvard Medical School
Assistant Psychiatrist
Massachusetts General Hospital
Boston, Massachusetts

Jonathan O. Cole, M.D.
Associate Professor of Psychiatry
Harvard Medical School
Boston, Massachusetts
Director, Psychopharmacology
  Section
Alcohol and Drug Abuse
  Research Center
McLean Hospital
Belmont, Massachusetts

C. Keith Conners, Ph.D.
Director of Developmental
  Neurobiology
Western Psychiatric Institute and
  Clinic
Professor of Psychiatry
University of Pittsburgh School
  of Medicine
Pittsburgh, Pennsylvania

Alberto DiMascio, Ph.D.
Director of Psychopharmacology
Department of Mental Health,
  Commonwealth of Massachusetts
Professor of Psychiatry
Tufts University School of
  Medicine
Boston, Massachusetts

Rachel Gittelman-Klein, Ph.D.
Director, Child Development Clinic
Long Island Jewish–Hillside
  Medical Center
Glen Oaks, New York
Associate Professor of Psychiatry
City University of New York
Queens College
Queens, New York

David J. Greenblatt, M.D.
Acting Chief, Clinical
  Pharmacology Unit
Massachusetts General Hospital
Assistant Professor of Medicine
Harvard Medical School
Boston, Massachusetts

Seymour S. Kety, M.D.
Director, Mailman Research Center
McLean Hospital
Belmont, Massachusetts
Professor of Psychiatry
Harvard Medical School
Boston, Massachusetts

Gerald L. Klerman, M.D.
Director, Stanley Cobb Psychiatric
  Research Laboratory
Massachusetts General Hospital
Professor of Psychiatry
Harvard Medical School
Boston, Massachusetts

John C. Kuehnle, M.D.
Clinical Director, Alcohol and
  Marihuana Research Unit
Alcohol and Drug Abuse Research
  Center
McLean Hospital
Belmont, Massachusetts
Assistant Professor of Psychiatry
Harvard Medical School
Boston, Massachusetts

Bernard Levy, M.D.
Medical Director
Human Resource Institute of
  Boston
Assistant Clinical Professor of
  Psychiatry
Harvard Medical School
Boston, Massachusetts

CONTENTS

PREFACE

Since the early 1950s, pharmacology and biochemistry have infused new life into psychiatry. Indeed, this field of clinical practice, which in the past moved away from the mainstream of medicine, is moving back, in large part as a consequence of the development of more effective pharmacologic therapies. Prior to the mid-twentieth century, chemical etiologies and treatments of psychiatric disorders were unproven and of limited clinical significance.

Many outstanding leaders in the early development of the field of psychiatry spoke of possible physiologic and biochemical etiologies and expressed interest and hope that the future would bring development of pharmacologic treatment of psychiatric disorders. Sigmund Freud himself was interested in psychopharmacology and conducted important studies of the psychoactive drug cocaine. Yet, paradoxically, many of Freud's more orthodox followers have been both reluctant to accept and slow to adopt pharmacologic treatment for their patients. Indeed, the early history of psychopharmacology has been punctuated by many disagreements and, frequently, unfriendly attitudes between psychoanalytically oriented psychiatrists and their more pharmacologically oriented colleagues. Fortunately for patients, this situation is improving greatly, and most practitioners in the mainstream of psychiatry are now more interested in learning about and employing drug therapy where it may be appropriate and potentially beneficial. Pharmacotherapy and psychotherapy are now seen by most professionals as complementary to each other rather than competitive or mutually exclusive.

In the current decade, sales of prescribed psychotropic drugs account for a significant proportion of total prescription drug sales, and most people have had some direct personal experience with prescribed psychoactive medicinals. Some prominent physicians claim that we are an overmedicated society; others feel that psychopharmacologic agents are being under prescribed. Irrespective of which side's contention may be closer to the truth, the situation today demands that all medical and mental health professionals become aware of the biologic and chemical aspects of the mechanisms and treatment of psychiatric disorders. It is not enough for physicians and psychiatrists alone to know about psychopharmacology; since many other professionals play important roles in the treatment of psychiatric patients, they too must attain a sophisticated grasp of this therapeutic modality.

A series of annual symposia on clinical psychopharmacology was organized under the sponsorship of the Human Resource Institute of Boston specifically for the purpose of aiding medical and mental health professionals in recognizing, diagnosing, and treating the various forms of psychiatric illness and of keeping them abreast of new developments in this field. This volume is a revised and updated presentation of selected lectures from the most recent of these symposia.

A work such as this is the result of many diverse contributions. I thank my parents and teachers for preparing me for the task, and my wife and children for sustaining and supporting me during its development. I owe a special debt of gratitude to my distinguished colleagues for their valuable contributions to this volume, especially to Dr. Bernard Levy for his continued stimulation and support. The help of my secretary, Louise Sloane, in organizing the symposia and preparing the manuscript is greatly appreciated. I also thank Margery Berube, managing editor of PSG Publishing Company, Inc., and Diane J. Neely, editor, who both did yeoman's service in keeping me on target and attending to all the details essential to bringing this work to fruition.

Jerrold G. Bernstein, M.D.
Newton Centre, Massachusetts

1 The Biological Bases of Mental Illness

Seymour S. Kety, M.D.

INTRODUCTION

Although schizophrenia, manic depression, and other forms of mental illness are not major causes of death, as are cancer or heart disease, they do rank with these as among our most serious national health problems. More than 10 million Americans experience one or more episodes of serious mental illness before they reach old age. The care of the mentally ill, inadequate as it often is, accounts for a major share of the budget of each of the 50 states; the national total is well over $5 billion annually. Less easily calculated is the human cost to those affected and their families.

Human disease in general is multifactorial; its origins are not found exclusively in the innate biological processes of the body or in environmental influences but in the continuing interaction between them. In the case of mental and behavioral disturbances, especially, this includes the important psychologic and social components of life experience which act together with biological and physical factors.

Biomedical research has been effective in the past in determining the biological bases of several serious forms of mental illness and in making their prevention possible. General paresis virtually disappeared as a cause of insanity in America once its syphilitic origin was established; similarly, pellagrous psychosis ceased to be a public health problem when it was found to be caused by a correctable dietary deficiency of nicotinic acid. But schizophrenia and manic-depressive illnesses have remained with us, and their seriousness is matched only by our ignorance regarding them. Since we do not yet know their causes or understand the processes through which they develop, we do not know how to prevent them. Their treatment, although improved dramatically through the use of recently discovered drugs, still leaves much to be desired. Over the past two decades, however, substantial research has indicated that these serious mental illnesses do have biochemical origins; and powerful new techniques and concepts have been developed which make the search for these causes more promising than ever before.

EARLY BIOLOGICAL APPROACHES

The idea of a biological basis for insanity is not new. The Hippocratic physicians of ancient Greece argued against the then-popular belief that insanity had supernatural causes: "... and by the same organ [the brain] we become mad and delirious and fears and terrors assail us. . . . All these things we endure from the brain, when it is not healthy but is more hot, more cold, more moist, or more dry than natural, or when it suffers any other preternatural and unusual affliction."[1]

The modern biochemical approach to mental illness can be traced to Thudichum, a physician and biochemist, who hypothesized nearly a century ago that many forms of insanity were the result of toxic substances fermented within the body, just as the psychosis of alcohol was caused by a toxic substance fermented outside. He received a research grant from the Privy Council in England that enabled him to spend 10 years examining this hypothesis. Significantly, Thudichum did not go to mental hospitals to examine the urine and blood of patients; instead he went to the slaughterhouse, obtained cattle brain, and began to study its normal chemical composition. It is very fortunate for us that he did because, in so doing, he laid the foundation of modern neurochemistry, which is the essential basis for studying the abnormal chemistry of the brain. If Thudichum had been less wise and courageous, or if the Parliament had been more insistent that he do "relevant" research, what contribution could he have made with the little knowledge that existed at that time? He would have frittered away the public funds and wasted 10 years of his life in a premature and futile search. By following the course he did, Thudichum was able to identify a large number of substances in the normal brain which were later found to be abnormal in a variety of neurological disorders.[2]

Fifty years ago biochemistry began to trace the complex processes of metabolism by which foodstuffs and oxygen are utilized and energy made available. This understanding was eventually applied to the brain—the brain's dependence on glucose was discovered and the oxygen utilized in various mental functions was measured. Many clinical states of mental abnormality were found to be associated with diminished oxygen consumption in the brain; these included senile psychosis, diabetic and other forms of coma, and a large variety of conditions in which there are clear, primary metabolic interferences with the energy utilization of the brain. These findings raised the hopes that other forms of mental illness might also have their roots in a simple deficiency of energy supply. Research soon showed, however, that a schizophrenic's brain uses exactly the same amount of oxygen as does the brain of a normal individual. Oxygen levels were also found to be unaffected in normal sleep, LSD psychosis, and the performance of mental arithmetic. The study of these four states led to a very important insight: the brain is qualitatively different from most other organs in the body. While the heart, the muscles, and the kidneys show a work output in relation to their energy utilization, the output of the brain cannot be measured in such simple terms. The brain uses the same amount of energy whether the individual is talking nonsense or speaking brilliant prose; it takes just as much oxygen to think an irrational thought as it does to think a rational one. It soon became clear that what mattered in mental functioning was not so much the supply of power to the brain as the way in which that energy was utilized later on.[3]

Once it was found that energy deficiencies were not the bases for the major psychoses, a number of other biochemical hypotheses were proposed. One hypothesis, developed 20 years ago, was that adrenaline was changed chemically in the blood of schizophrenics to a substance called adrenochrome, thought at one time to be hallucinogenic. This hypothesis encouraged Julius Axelrod to elucidate the normal pathways of catecholamine metabolism in the body and brain. His fundamental contributions here provided an important base for much of current research. When the metabolism of adrenaline in schizophrenics was examined, however, no evidence for adrenochrome formation could be found. Other chemical theories of schizophrenia abounded;[4] the disease was ascribed by some to the presence of particular psychotogenic proteins in the blood, described by some as "taraxein," by others as "S-protein." These claims were not confirmed. In retrospect, the difficulty with the theories proposed at that time is quite obvious. These heroic efforts were simply premature. They were attempting to bridge the great gap between existing biochemical knowledge and mental illness in one span, before the foundations had been laid. The numerous "breakthroughs" that turned out to be illusory contributed to a disparagement of biology in the field of mental illness and a conviction that those disorders were primarily psychological and social problems.

In the absence of credible biochemical findings pertinent to schizophrenia and manic-depressive illness, observations suggesting their hereditary nature became crucial. Clear evidence that these illnesses had important genetic bases would justify a continued search for biochemical causes, since genetic factors can express themselves only through biochemical process.

THE GENETICS OF SCHIZOPHRENIA AND MANIC-DEPRESSIVE ILLNESS

The evidence for genetic factors in the major mental illnesses was compelling but not conclusive, since factors other than genetic ones could account for the observations that were available. Psychiatrists had known for a long time (and every epidemiological study has confirmed the observation) that these illnesses run in families. There is approximately a 10% risk for the occurrence of schizophrenia in the parents, siblings, and children of schizophrenic patients, and manic-depressive illness shows a comparable familial tendency. Although this is compatible with the theory of genetic transmission, it is by no means proof of it. Health and poverty run in families too but are not genetically transmitted; and the familial occurrence of pellagra once permitted a belief in the genetic nature of what we now know to be primarily a nutritional disorder. Members of a family share not only their genetic endowment but also their environment, and either or both of these factors may be responsible for familial disorders. In addition, the study of the familial occurrence of mental illness poses some special difficulties. First, there is the problem of ascertainment and selective bias. If there are more people with serious mental illness than are known to psychiatrists, then it stands to reason that a family with two cases has a greater chance of being discovered than a family with only one. There is, therefore, a built-in bias in favor of finding familial forms of mental illness. A second problem is the obvious subjective bias involved in diagnosis. Schizophrenia is not a disorder diagnosed by blood tests or x-ray findings, but is a collection of subjectively evaluated symptoms. A diagnosis of schizophrenia represents an opinion on the part of psychiatrists that a patient has enough of these symptoms to be considered schizophrenic. And although subjective evaluation can be very sensitive, it is also easily influenced by preconceived notions and irrelevant information.

For many years, the best evidence for the importance of genetic factors in mental illness came from studies of the twins of schizophrenic and manic-depressive individuals. These studies have generally shown a high incidence of schizophrenia among the identical twins of schizophrenics and a low incidence among their fraternal twins; similar results have been obtained for the manic-depressive psychoses. These findings are compatible with genetic theories since identical twins share all their genetic endowment while fraternal twins are no closer genetically than are ordinary siblings. In the last 15 years, twin studies have been able to avoid ascertainment and subjective bias and still find the same results. But because these studies could not control environmental factors, they did not provide conclusive evidence for genetic transmission. Identical twins share more of their environment than do fraternal twins. They usually live together and sleep together, their parents parade them in the same perambulator and dress them alike, they have the same friends and experiences. Unless one could randomize their environment, one couldn't be sure to what extent the shared psychosis in identical twins was due to ego identification, mimicry, or other environmental factors they shared in addition to their genetics. There must have been loopholes in the genetic evidence large enough that whole schools of psychiatry could march through, denying that mental illness had any genetic or biological basis.

Over the past 15 years, however, a new approach has been used which appears to have succeeded in separating genetic factors from environmental factors in the transmission of schizophrenia. This consists of the study of adopted individuals, who share their genetic endowment with their biological relatives, but share their environment with their adoptive relatives. In the several studies which have been completed to date the results are quite consistent. Schizophrenia continues to run in families, but now its high prevalence is restricted to the biological relatives of schizophrenic adoptees with whom they share genetic, but few, if any, environmental factors. The adoptive relatives of schizophrenics, who reared them and shared their environment, show no more tendency to schizophrenia than does the population at large.[5] [6]

This is stronger evidence than that previously available, but not conclusive because adoptees are not separated at the time of conception. They share nine months of in utero environment and a minimum of a few days of infancy with their biological mothers; in those interactions it is not impossible that nongenetic influences may be acquired that could produce schizophrenia years later. But even that possibility can be ruled out. The biological parents of adopted individuals are usually young and fertile; they have many other children, often with different partners. This is especially true for the biological fathers, so that adoptees have a large number of paternal half-siblings who did not have the same mother and shared none of the environment—in utero, neonatal, or postnatal—with the adoptee.

When the half-siblings of schizophrenic adoptees and of normal control adoptees were examined for schizophrenia (by procedures designed to protect against subjective and ascertainment bias), the results were striking. Schizophrenia was significantly concentrated in the paternal half-siblings of the schizophrenic adoptees while the half-siblings of the controls showed the same low prevalence found in the general population. This constitutes the most definitive evidence to date for the operation of genetic factors in the transmission of schizophrenia.[6]

Studies using adopted populations have not yet been completed for manic and depressive illnesses. However, there have been two reports recently of the occurrence in certain families of manic-depressive illness in association with traits (such as color blindness and a specific blood group) that are known to be controlled by genes in the X chromosome. Although this association does not occur in all families with these disorders, where it does occur, it suggests an X-linked genetic transmission.[6]

Taken together, these studies force one to the conclusion that genetic factors play a crucial etiological role in the majority of patients with typical schizophrenia and in a number of manic-depressive illnesses.[6] But this is not the only evidence that justifies a continued and augmented search for the biological substrates of mental illness.

CHEMICAL SYNAPSES AND PSYCHOPHARMACOLOGY

While the nature:nurture controversy was going on, those equipped to study the fundamental processes of the brain had not been idle. During the past 25 years there has been a dramatic growth in the neurosciences and an unprecedented development of knowledge regarding the brain and behavior. One of the breakthroughs that occurred, with special pertinence to psychiatry, was the recognition and demonstration of chemical transmission at the synapse, the highly specialized junction between nerve cells through which information is carried.

Previously, the brain had been thought of as a highly complex electrical computer. While the ultimate energy source for this computer was known to be biochemical, involving the utilization of oxygen and glucose, it was widely believed that the "wiring" of the computer itself was electrical rather than chemical in nature. The discovery of chemical synapses changed this picture radically. It became evident that the brain was different from any machine which had ever been devised by man; it was a computer in which the billions of switches were not electrical, but chemical switches which were turned on and off by biochemical processes. Sensory processing, perception, the storage and retrieval of information, thought, feeling, and behavior all depended upon the operation of these chemical switches. This discovery finally indicated the sites at which chemical substances, metabolic products, hormones, and drugs could modify these crucial aspects of mental state and behavior. If there are biochemical disturbances in mental illness, they could be expected to have effects at the synapses; and drugs which ameliorate these illnesses should exert their influence there as well.[7][8]

Although there may be hundreds of billions of synapses in the human brain, they are organized in a marvelously systematic way along certain pathways that are being mapped by neuroanatomists. Scientists have identified several types of neurotransmitters (chemical substances responsible for the transmission of signals between synapses) and have found these different substances to be associated with different pathways, functions, and behavioral states. The catecholamine transmitters adrenaline, noradrenaline, and dopamine were first identified in the adrenal gland and in the peripheral sympathetic nervous system. They are now known to be important neurotransmitters in the brain, where they appear to be involved in emotional states such as arousal, rage, fear, pleasure, motivation, and exhilaration. Serotonin, first discovered in the intestine, has also been identified in the brain, where it seems to play a crucial role in sleep and wakefulness, in certain types of sexual activity, and perhaps in modulating, damping, and balancing a wide range of synaptic activity that we are only beginning to understand. Acetylcholine, which is known to be the transmitter between nerve and muscle and is therefore crucial to every voluntary movement, has also been found to be involved in a very large proportion of brain synapses. There are neurotransmitters such as gamma-aminobutyric acid, and certain other amino acids and polypeptides, which have been discovered more recently; undoubtedly many more remain to be found. Fundamental knowledge of the synapse and chemical neurotransmission has important implications for the understanding and treatment of nervous and mental disease and represents an area of unusual promise for the future.

While noradrenaline and serotonin were being identified in the brain, it was discovered quite independently, and almost accidentally, that several drugs exert important effects on mood. The first of these was reserpine, which was known to be useful in the treatment of hypertension. In a small percentage of patients, reserpine produced a state of depression very much like the clinical one known to psychiatrists. At the same time, scientists at the National Heart Institute made the imporant discovery that reserpine caused a decrease in levels of serotonin and noradrenaline in the brain.[4][9]

A few years later a new drug, iproniazid, was shown to be highly effective in the treatment of tuberculosis. When it was found to cause emotional excitement in some patients, it was supplanted by other drugs equally effective and without such side effects. But this strange side effect of iproniazid, while a hazard in the treatment of tuberculosis, became the basis for an effective treatment of depression.[9] Iproniazid was discovered to block the enzyme monoamine oxidase, which is responsible for inactivating serotonin and the catecholamines. Thus, iproniazid enhanced the effect of these transmitters, an action opposite to that of reserpine. A number of other drugs were developed which were also monoamine oxidase inhibitors and effective in the treatment of depression. Even more effective were the tricyclic antidepressants, including the drugs imipramine and amitriptyline, which enhance the synaptic actions of noradrenaline and serotonin by a mechanism other than monoamine oxidase inhibitors.[8] Electroshock therapy is effective in the treatment of patients with some kinds of severe depression, and it is interesting that administering similar shocks to experimental animals also increases the levels of noradrenaline and serotonin in their brains.

The foregoing observations suggest that clinical depression may be the result of an inadequacy of noradrenaline or serotonin (or both) at particular synapses in the brain, and, similarly, that mania, the obverse of depression, may represent an overactivity of these synapses. The testing of this hypothesis has engaged a number of research groups. Certain types of depression and mania have been found to be associated with a decrease or an increase, respectively, of a particular breakdown product of noradrenaline in the urine; this substance appears to be derived largely from noradrenaline in the brain. Others, examining the cerebrospinal fluid, have found evidence of a decrease in serotonin metabolism in the brains of patients suffering from manic or depressive psychosis. A very effective agent in the treatment of mania and in the prevention of manic-depressive illness is lithium, a relatively simple ion closely related to sodium (which plays a crucial role in synaptic function); lithium appears to increase the synaptic levels of serotonin. Clearly there is much work which can be done to pursue these interesting leads.

In 1950 a drug was developed which was found to be more effective than any previous treatment in the relief of the major symptoms of schizophrenia.[10] This action was discovered in an interesting and unexpected manner. Pharmacologists had been developing and studying drugs which blocked the action of histamine, an endogenous substance which appears to play an important role in many forms of allergy. One of these drugs also blocked the activity of the sympathetic nervous system. Laborit, a French anesthesiologist, had been looking for a drug which had such properties for use in the prevention of surgical shock, reasoning that both histamine and sympathetic overactivity might contribute to shock in surgical operations. He used this drug in preoperative medication and, through careful observations, noted that it produced in his patients an unexpected sedation. This sedation was different from that known to occur with the barbiturates; Laborit described it as a "euphoric quietude." He felt that such an effect might be helpful in the treatment of disturbed patients, and suggested this to some psychiatrists. The drug used by Laborit was the immediate forerunner of chlorpromazine, which revolutionized the treatment of schizophrenia.[10]

Chlorpromazine was immediately seized upon and used throughout the civilized world because it was different from any previous treatment for schizophrenia. While this new drug quieted schizophrenics, it did not act like a tranquilizer; its action was much more specific. Not only would it quiet a disturbed and aggressive schizophrenic patient, it would also attenuate his hallucinations and delusions, and sometimes reduce his apathy. No sedative ever discovered had all of those beneficial effects. Here at last was a substance which appeared to be acting almost specifically upon the behavioral and cognitive features that characterized schizophrenia.[10]

In addition to its therapeutic effects in schizophrenia, however, chlorpromazine had an important side effect; it produced in some patients the facial and motor disturbances which are seen in Parkinson's disease. Modifications of chlorpromazine were developed in an effort to preserve the therapeutic benefit while avoiding this drawback, but, with very few exceptions, all the effective agents found also had this side effect. In addition to chlorpromazine and its derivatives (known collectively as phenothiazines), an entirely new chemical class of drugs appeared, the butyrophenones, which was also effective in the treatment of schizophrenia but suffered as well from the tendency to produce symptoms of parkinsonism. It appeared that the side effect was intimately related to the therapeutic action, but for 10 years no explanation of either was possible.

In 1960, a new technique was developed in Sweden for identifying certain neurotransmitters within the brain by means of their characteristic fluorescence under appropriate conditions. That technique was quickly applied by neuroanatomists and used to trace circuits within the brain which utilized these transmitters. The nigro-striatal pathway, which was known to be damaged in patients with true Parkinson's disease, was found to use dopamine as a transmitter. This led to the hypothesis and the ultimate demonstration that a partial destruction of the dopamine-synthesizing nerve cells was the basis for Parkinson's disease. Efforts to replenish the lost dopamine by administration of its precursor L-dopa were successful, leading to marked improvement in the patients; this represented one of the major contributions of fundamental research to the treatment of neurologic illness in recent years.

These remarkable findings also had an important impact on psychiatry. It was suggested first by Arvid Carlsson that the antipsychotic drugs must act by blocking the effects of dopamine in the brain, since this would explain their tendency to produce the symptoms of Parkinson's disease. On the basis of his studies and more recent observations on dopamine synapses in the brain and on the components of such synapses studied in vitro, it is now clear that Carlsson's insight was correct.[11] A major action of both the phenothiazine and the butyrophenone drugs is to block the dopamine synapses within the brain.

The drug amphetamine also affects dopamine synapses, but amphetamine exaggerates the effects of dopamine instead of diminishing them. Clinically, too, amphetamine can be considered the direct opposite of the antipsychotic drugs. In animals it produces stereotypic movements of various kinds and aimless pacing, behavior patterns also seen in schizophrenia. When amphetamine is abused by human subjects, it produces a psychosis which is often indistinguishable from schizophrenia, and the same drugs which are effective in the treatment of schizophrenia are also specific in terminating an amphetamine psychosis. Amphetamine is also known to exacerbate the psychosis of schizophrenic individuals.[9]

The overall picture is very clear: drugs which enhance dopamine activity in the brain tend to produce or aggravate schizophrenic symptoms, while those which diminish dopamine activity are capable of relieving those symptoms.[12]

These findings do not necessarily indicate that schizophrenia is caused by an overactivity of dopamine synapses. One hypothesis does hold that the disorder is due to an excess of dopamine, stemming perhaps from a deficiency in the enzyme responsible for converting dopamine to noradrenaline; but there are several other possibilities. Dopamine-containing neurons interact with many other neurotransmitters and neurohormones in the brain. For example, dopamine inhibits the release of the hormone prolactin from the pituitary gland; the phenothiazines, by blocking the effects of dopamine, have been shown to raise levels of prolactin throughout the bloodstream and in the cerebrospinal fluid. The activity of dopamine pathways is also affected by neural circuits that use acetylcholine, serotonin, and gamma-aminobutyric acid, and it could be these substances that are more directly related to schizophrenic symptoms. But whatever the reasons for the therapeutic effects of the antipsychotic drugs, it is clear that continued and expanded research on dopamine and other neurotransmitters, on their distribution and synaptic activity, and on the interrelationships of these neurotransmitters with behavior at very basic as well as clinical levels will contribute to our understanding of these illnesses.[12] With this understanding will certainly come more specific treatments for these illnesses and, ultimately, a means of preventing them.

Other chemical substances besides the catecholamines have also been implicated in schizophrenia, though the evidence for their role in the disease is much less clear. Several drugs, such as mescaline, LSD, and dimethyltryptamine (DMT), are capable of inducing hallucinations and some of the other symptoms of schizophrenia and have, to some, suggested hypotheses about the nature of schizophrenia itself. Mescaline and dimethyltryptamine chemically resemble substances normally present in the body, but modified by the addition of methyl (CH_3) groups. Shortly after the elucidation of biological transmethylation, by which such groups are added to particular molecules, it was suggested that this normal process might be disturbed in schizophrenia, so that abnormal methylated compounds with hallucinogenic properties might accumulate in the brain. This hypothesis received some support from the finding that the amino acid methionine, which can serve as a donor of methyl groups, tends to exacerbate psychotic symptoms in schizophrenic patients. More recently, several groups of researchers have detected an enzyme in the lung and brain of animals and man which is capable of methylating substances normally present in the brain, such as tryptamine, thus converting them to hallucinogenic substances like dimethyltryptamine.[13] In some laboratories, such methylated compounds have been found in the body fluids of schizophrenic patients. These findings, if confirmed, would suggest a link between schizophrenia and the presence of metabolically synthesized dimethyltryptamine or other hallucinogens.

In addition to inactivating serotonin and the catecholamines in the normal brain, monoamine oxidase has the ability to destroy many other amines, including dimethyltryptamine. It is possible that the methylating enzyme present in the normal brain is constantly producing hallucinogenic products that are normally detoxified by monoamine oxidase; if that enzyme were deficient in schizophrenics, these hallucinogens could accumulate. Recently, several groups have found that the blood platelets of schizophrenics are indeed low in this enzyme.[14] Especially interesting was the finding that relatives of schizophrenics, especially identical twins, showed this enzyme deficiency, although they may not have been schizophrenic themselves. Clearly, this has potential relevance to the genetic factors that may predispose an individual to developing schizophrenia. At present, however, some laboratories have failed to confirm these findings in platelets and no one has demonstrated a deficiency of this enzyme in the brain.

Whether or not methylated hallucinogenic amines accumulate in schizophrenia is still a matter of controversy. But, the finding that all of us have the capability of forming hallucinogenic substances in our bodies and brains is a striking observation that must be further explored.

Today the number of new techniques waiting to be applied to the problems of mental illness is legion. There are the techniques that identify and localize specific neurotransmitters and enzymes by means of induced fluorescence. There are procedures employing radioactive tracers that permit one to map the circuits of the brain. Cell culture techniques have made possible the identification of genetic metabolic errors in a substantial number of medical and neurologic illnesses. There are sophisticated genetic studies that permit the localization of these defects to particular chromosomes. A number of hitherto obscure medical and neurologic illnesses have been found to result from slow virus infestation; and recent advances in virology may uncover similar causes for the mental illnesses as well. Neurobiology and neuropharmacology supply powerful tools for the study of the synapse, which has already led to an elucidation of drug action and to the development of safer and more effective drugs. There are chemical analytical techniques, such as the mass spectrograph, which make possible the discovery and quantification of infinitesimal amounts of abnormal chemical substances in various body fluids. Rigorous and quantifiable behavioral techniques clarify the relationships of the biological mechanisms to behavior, bringing them to bear upon a wide variety of mental processes, such as cognition, learning, motivation and mood.

A new generation of neuroscientists has been trained, skilled in fundamental research and highly motivated to apply these techniques in unravelling the mysteries of the brain. The time has never been more propitious for progress toward an understanding of the serious disturbances of the human mind.

REFERENCES

1. Adams, F. (trans. and ed.): *The Genuine Works of Hippocrates*. Baltimore: The Williams & Wilkins Co., 1939.

2. Thudichum, J.W.L.: *A Treatise on the Chemical Constitution of the Brain*. London: Bailliere, Tindall and Cox, 1884.

3. Kety, S.S.: Relationship between energy metabolism of the brain and functional activity. In Kety, S.S., Everts, E.V., and Williams, H.L. (eds): *Sleep and Altered States of Consciousness*, Res. Publ. Assoc. Nerv. Ment. Dis., Vol. XLV. Baltimore: The Williams & Wilkins Co., 1967, pp. 39-45.

4. Kety, S.S.: Biochemical theories of schizophrenia. A two-part critical review of current theories and of the evidence used to support them. *Science* 129: 1528-1532, 1590-1596, 1959.

5. Rosenthal, D. and Kety, S.S. (eds.): *The Transmission of Schizophrenia*. Oxford: Pergamon Press, 1968.

6. Fieve, R., Rosenthal, D., and Brill, H. (eds.): *Genetic Research in Psychiatry*. Baltimore: Johns Hopkins University Press, 1975.

7. Matthysse, S.: Antipsychotic drug actions: a clue to the neuropathology of schizophrenia? *Fed. Proc.* 32:200-205, 1973.

8. Matthysse, S. and Pope, A.: The approach to schizophrenia through molecular pathology. In Good, R.A., Day, S.B., and Yunis, J.J. (eds.): *Molecular Pathology*. Springfield, Ill: Charles C. Thomas, 1975, pp. 744-763.

9. Klein, D.F. and Davis, J.M.: *Diagnosis and Drug Treatment of Psychiatric Disorders*. Baltimore: The Williams & Wilkins Co., 1969.

10. Swazey, J.P.: *Chlorpromazine in Psychiatry, A Study of Therapeutic Innovation*. Cambridge, Mass: MIT Press, 1974.

11. Carlsson, A. and Lindqvist, M.: Effect of chlorpromazine or haloperidol on formation of 3-methoxytyramine and normetanephrine in mouse brain. *Acta Physiol. et Toxicol.* 20:140, 1973.

12. Matthysse, S. and Kety, S.S. (eds.): *Catecholamines and Schizophrenia*. Oxford: Pergamon Press, 1975.

13. Saavedra, J.M., Coyle, J.T., and Axelrod, J.: The distribution and properties of the non-specific N-methyltransferase in brain. *J. Neurochem.* 20:743-752, 1973.

14. Wyatt, R.J., Murphy, D.L., Belmaker, R. et al: Reduced monoamine oxidase activity in platelets: a possible genetic marker for vulnerability to schizophrenia. *Science* 179:916, 1973.

2 The Clinical Use of Antianxiety Drugs

Jonathan O. Cole, M.D.

Anxiety is a term widely invoked in psychiatry to explain all manner of clinical phenomena. From the pharmacologic standpoint, it makes a substantial difference whether anxiety symptoms commonly associated with free-floating or unfocused anxiety—apprehension, fear, jitteriness, nervousness—occur relatively independently of other phenomena or whether they occur in a context of depression, psychosis, or organic brain syndrome. It is also pharmacologically useful to distinguish (1) anticipatory anxiety—anxiety experienced in anticipation of a stressful, painful, or unpleasant event; (2) phobic anxiety—unreasonable anxiety or apprehension associated with some specific external situation or object; (3) panic anxiety—discrete, acute, severe episodes of panic occurring without discernible outside cause; and (4) chronic anxiety—a constant state of dysphoria characterized by nervousness, anxiety irritability, and related symptoms.[1] In addition, it is probably reasonable to distinguish autonomic manifestations of anxiety (e.g., palpitations, sweating, dizziness, irregular heart rhythm, abdominal distress, tremor, dry mouth), which may sometimes occur independently of the subjective feelings of anxiety or may cause the subjective feelings of anxiety.

14

Unfortunately, almost all the reported clinical trials to evaluate the efficacy of antianxiety drugs in man have disregarded these distinctions and tend to include in the study all patients who seek medical help for complaints of "anxiety." Further, the most common self-report instruments and therapist's rating instruments used in outpatient studies of anxiety include a variety of anxiety symptoms covering subjective experience of anxiety and autonomic sequelae of anxiety in about equal proportions. Other neurotic symptoms—for example, obsessive thinking, compulsive behavior, and symptoms reflecting irritability, anger, depression, and concentration difficulty— are also often included in such scales. To make matters worse, in most heterogeneous outpatient populations, depressive symptoms and anxiety symptoms often coexist, making it very difficult to derive from such multi-item rating scales any factor which reflects pure anxiety; more commonly anxiety and depression items load on the same factor.

AVAILABLE ANTIANXIETY DRUGS

Historically, the earliest antianxiety drugs were alcohol and opium. Alcohol has never been specifically studied in a controlled fashion as a treatment for common outpatient anxiety. However, the drug is widely self-prescribed to control social anxiety, probably of an anticipatory sort, and at low doses it is probably effective. Opium and related drugs have the joint properties of analgesia and anxiety relief, the latter probably achieved through the production of mild euphoria. The abuse liability of both classes of drugs precludes their use as antianxiety agents in clinical medicine except in highly unusual situations. There is evidence, for example, that alcohol in low doses improves mood and social adjustment of geriatric-psychiatric patients in institutional settings;[2] and opiates are frequently used as preoperative medication to decrease apprehension.

In the late 1800s bromide salts were widely used as antianxiety agents, but they have lost prominence in clinical therapy because of their long half-lives in the body and their tendency to accumulate and produce bromide psychosis. The older sedative-hypnotic antianxiety agents, other than the bromides, are the barbiturates (which exist in wide variety), chloral hydrate, and paraldehyde. Paraldehyde's foul taste and pervasive odor have relegated it to a role only in the treatment of alcohol withdrawal states and occasional medical situations, but even here its use is declining.[3]

Prior to 1950 there appeared a variety of nonbarbiturate hypnotics and sedatives: primarily, glutethimide(Doriden), methyprylon(Noludar), and ethchlorvynol (Placidyl).[4] All these drugs have been used chiefly as hypnotics to relieve insomnia, but all can be used in lower doses to induce daytime sedation and relieve anxiety. Unfortunately, the early hope that these nonbarbiturate agents would be safer drugs than the barbiturates, which they were designed to replace, has proved to be totally without foundation. These drugs have equally lethal potential and, at least in the case of glutethimide, may be more lethal than the short-acting barbiturates. They have equal abuse liability and have no discernible special value in either the treatment of anxiety or the relief of insomnia.

Meprobamate (Equanil), which first came to general medical attention about 1957, occupies a position between the barbiturates which preceded it and the benzodiazepines which succeeded it, and is probably somewhat better at relieving anxiety than the barbiturates and somewhat safer in terms of abuse liability and lethality when taken in suicide attempts. The benzodiazepines, diazepam (Valium) chlordiazepoxide (Librium), oxazepam (Serax), and clorazepate (Tranxene), are all probably safer, more effective, and more broadly useful than the barbiturates or the other antianxiety and hypnotic drugs which preceded them, though they still have their problems.[5]

All of these drugs—the barbiturates, the nonbarbiturate sedatives, and the benzodiazepines—are usefully classed together by Hollister as sedative L-hypnotic antianxiety agents.[6] Two somewhat newer members of the group deserve special mention. These are tybamate (Tybatran), a short-acting drug somewhat similar chemically to meprobamate, and methaqualone (Quaalude), a recent sedative-hypnotic of no particular advantage relative to the barbiturates. Methaqualone simply underlines the fact that history repeats itself. It first became available approximately 10 years ago and was judged to be safer and better than other hypnotics until a rash of reports on its abuse liability served to reemphasize the fact that drugs in this general class are unlikely to be totally abuse-free. Tybamate is the only drug, to date, to challenge this presumption. It has been impossible to induce physical dependence on tybamate in either dogs or man.

Hollister's second category of antianxiety agents is that of the autonomic-sedative antianxiety drugs.[6] Currently, the most widely used member of this class is hydroxyzine (Atarax, Vistaril), a sedative antihistamine which is marketed for use in anxiety. Diphenhydramine (Benadryl) also has some sedative-hypnotic properties and is sometimes used for this purpose. As will be noted below, the tricyclic antidepressants can be used as antianxiety agents and when so used would fall within this classification.

Propranolol (Inderal) probably deserves separate classification. It is an autonomic agent without appreciable central sedative properties;

it appears to have a selective action on somatic components of anxiety.[7] When promazine (Phenergan), an antihistaminic phenothiazine, and the other antipsychotic phenothiazines are used in low doses to produce mild sedation and relieve anxiety, they also belong properly under this general rubric.

PHARMACOLOGY

It is fascinating to note that 25 years ago the catecholamines would have been considered the obvious agents which cause anxiety. It is therefore noteworthy that over the last 20 years catecholamines have been frequently invoked to explain depression and schizophrenia, but rarely invoked in theories of anxiety or in attempts to explain the mechanisms of action of antianxiety drugs. Recently, Stein and Wise have put forward the general theory that oxazepam, as a representative benzodiazepine, acts by decreasing norepinephrine turnover and serotonin turnover.[8] The norepinephrine effect is short lasting, while the serotonin effect is long lasting. They therefore hypothesize that the norepinephrine effect of oxazepam is related to its short-acting hypnotic action and the serotonin effect is related to its longer-acting antianxiety effect. However, Cook has recently presented evidence that the norepinephrine effect only occurs with the initial dose of a benzodiazepine and is never seen again when the dose is readministered even a week or two later,[9] which casts doubt on the generality of the phenomenon described by Stein and Wise. The serotonin effect may well have some relevance to the antianxiety action of these drugs, but its role is still somewhat unclear.

The benzodiazepines have other biochemical effects.[9] They act to stimulate gamma-aminobutyric acid (GABA) synapses, an action which is blocked when GABA levels have been reduced by an inhibitor of GABA synthesis. This effect is, unfortunately, probably unrelated to the antianxiety effects of the agents and is more likely to play a role in their anticonvulsant and muscle relaxant properties. Snyder has recently emphasized the fact that benzodiazepines compete for glycine receptors on the neurons in the central nervous system.[10] According to Cook, these effects do not correlate well with the drugs' antianxiety properties and again may well be irrelevant to the mechanism of action of these drugs in anxiety. The effects of these agents as phosphodiesterase inhibitors are also probably irrelevant to their antianxiety action.

We are therefore left with a group of drugs with proven efficacy in relieving clinical anxiety and in relieving insomnia, and we have not yet found any clear biochemical mechanism of action relevant to these effects. These drugs, as well as the barbiturates and propranolol, do increase beta activity in the human electroencephalogram, but again the relevance of this effect to anxiety relief is obscure.

Irwin has studied the effects of the sedative-hypnotics and of the autonomic antianxiety compounds on animal behavior, using a somewhat clinical, "mental status" model.[11] He observes that the sedative-hypnotics in general increase exploratory behavior and motor activity at low doses. They tend to augment the animal's response to environmental stimuli, while the antipsychotic drugs tend to reduce this response. In man, the antipsychotic drugs decrease exploratory behavior and motor activity while presumably still relieving anxiety. Irwin infers that drugs such as diazepam should be most useful in patients in whom the goal is increased activity and social interaction, and that the antipsychotic drugs should be most useful in patients in whom decreased motor activity and social interaction is sought. His inference—that diazepam would be more useful in inhibited, anxious neurotics, while a phenothiazine would be more useful in anxious impulse disorders and in agitated schizophrenics and depressions—does in fact fit the known clinical actions of these drugs. However, his hypothesis has never been directly tested in more conventional anxious outpatients, where such distinctions probably could be usefully made.

The most useful screening technique for new sedative-hypnotic antianxiety agents is one which involves drug-induced disinhibition of conditioned suppression of behavior in animals. A thirsty animal is trained to press a lever to receive a water reward. He is then exposed periodically to a condition in which a special light is kept on. The animal receives a painful shock to his feet if he presses the lever for water during this time and learns to stop pressing the lever while the light is on. This effect of the light and the shock is known as "conditioned suppression." At appropriate doses, benzodiazepines, alcohol, and barbiturates all cause the animal to go ahead and press the lever anyway, even in the presence of the light and the foot shock.[9] Since analgesic opiates do not have this effect, this action is presumed not to be mediated through analgesia. Interestingly, no other class of psychoactive drug in clinical use has this effect in general, although Cook reports that trifluoperazine in very low doses has some action of this sort,[9] a finding which correlates well with the utility of antipsychotic drugs in very low doses in the treatment of outpatient anxiety. In terms of the classes of anxiety noted in the beginning of this chapter, this effect would be an example of drug alleviation of anticipatory anxiety.

Most of the antianxiety drugs, whether sedative-hypnotic or autonomic-sedative, will demonstrate a taming effect at some dose in angry rhesus monkeys. Whether this effect is in fact related to anxiety relief is obscure.

The sedative-hypnotics tend to raise the convulsive threshold and are usually effective treatments of alcohol withdrawal or barbiturate withdrawal when used in appropriate doses at appropriate intervals. Antipsychotic drugs tend to lower the convulsive threshold.[3]

EFFICACY OF ANTIANXIETY DRUGS

Previous review papers have gone over this area in more detail.[1 5 6 12] To summarize the matter briefly, there is overwhelming evidence that the benzodiazepines chlordiazepoxide, diazepam, and oxazepam are clearly and significantly more effective than placebo in treating outpatient anxiety. Over 80% of the published controlled studies comparing these drugs with placebo bear this out. The barbiturates and meprobamate, however, tend to be somewhat less effective, being shown to be superior to placebo in only two thirds of published studies. However, the technology for doing such trials has improved in the last 10 to 15 years, and perhaps some of the reported lower efficacy of the barbiturates and meprobamate is due to the fact that they were studied with older, less sophisticated research methods. As an example of this, tybamate, which may well not be an exceptionally effective drug, is shown to be superior to placebo in 15 of 16 published studies.[5]

Controlled studies directly comparing benzodiazepines with older antianxiety drugs such as meprobamate and the barbiturates produce less clear results, though the benzodiazepines are usually somewhat superior. On the other hand, occasional large scale, well-designed, controlled studies of antianxiety drugs fail to show much evidence of drug superiority over placebo. A Veterans Administration collaborative study of chlordiazepoxide vs placebo is a case in point. In this eight-week study, chlordiazepoxide was clearly superior to placebo only at the five-week rating point.[13]

Rickels and Wheatley have produced evidence to suggest that in patients whose anxiety is of relatively short duration, the placebo response is so high (around 80%) that it equals, or even slightly surpasses, the efficacy of antianxiety drugs. On the other hand, in more chronic patients in the same studies, the efficacy of the antianxiety drug remained at about 70% to 80%, while placebo response dropped to about 20%.[14 15]

In a large series of studies of a variety of drugs used in outpatient psychiatry, Rickels has consistently shown that the drug-placebo difference is greatest in patients being treated in the offices of general practitioners.[12] The drug-placebo difference is somewhat decreased in lower economic class, clinic patients studied in urban, general hospital outpatient clinics and is often almost nonexistent in patients studied in the office practices of psychiatrists. These studies do not permit firm conclusions to be drawn about the reasons for the discrepancies, but one can assume that psychiatrists tend to see the more seriously ill patients who have often failed to respond to antianxiety drug treatment provided by primary care physicians. Poverty clinic patients often have a major focus on somatic symptoms and tend to be more liable to somatic side effects when under a wide range of drug therapies, and this may interfere with their clinical response.

Studies of antianxiety drugs in symptomatic volunteers—individuals with anxiety at least as severe as that found in psychiatric outpatients, who respond to advertisements to participate in antianxiety drug studies—show that this population is also very sensitive to drug-placebo differences. This is perhaps attributable to the high level of cooperation generally encountered with paid symptomatic volunteers and possibly to the generally higher level of intelligence and motivation often found in such individuals.

A large and growing literature exists on predictors of clinical response to antianxiety agents in nonpsychotic psychiatric outpatients. In his most recent review, Rickels summarizes the situation by presenting data derived from predictor analyses of over 400 outpatients treated with the benzodiazepines chlordiazepoxide or diazepam.[12] Patients who respond best to these drugs are characteristically employed, married, treated in a family practice setting, better educated, expecting drug treatment, and aware that they have emotional problems. In making his initial evaluation of such patients, the physician feels that they have a good prognosis; he feels comfortable with such patients; and he feels comfortable in prescribing drugs for them. The illness presented by "good prognosis" patients is of acute duration. The patients have had relatively little exposure to drugs in the prior treatment of their anxiety; they have had a good response to the drugs they have received; they lack current medical illness; and they show sedative side effects after two weeks of treatment and are diagnosed as anxiety reactions or mixed anxiety-depression reactions. Patients responding well to these drugs generally present with a history of a precipitating stress. Females who respond well to these drugs are generally not in the menopause and have not had a hysterectomy.

On the Hopkins Symptom Checklist, a multi-item self-report form, patients responding well to these drugs tend to be more symptomatic on the anxiety factor and to show less psychopathology in the areas of depression, interpersonal sensitivity, and obsessive-compulsive symptoms.[16] In a reanalysis of his extensive fund of data from a variety of studies, Rickels also observes that the degree of symptom relief obtained in anxious outpatients receiving these benzodiazepines is relatively modest.[12] The effect is clearly superior to that obtained by placebo, but at the end of therapy the patients still show considerable residual symptomatology and resemble a sample of patients referred by their primary care physicians for significant emotional problems. They do not achieve the low level of self-reported symptomatology characteristic of general practice patients who are judged by their treating physicians to not have any appreciable emotional pathology. The benzodiazepines are therefore ameliorative rather than curative.

Rickels has also gone to considerable trouble to carry out a study on a drug preparation essentially identical to Compoz, an over-the-counter antianxiety agent. His studies showed this drug to be no more effective than inert placebo.

Given the extensive review of the efficacy data on all antianxiety agents now on the market in this country, it is safe to assume that other marketed drugs, such as hydroxyzine and tybamate, are also significantly more effective than placebo in general clinical use. Although the tricyclic antidepressant drugs have been studied almost exclusively in outpatients presenting with mixed anxiety and depression, doxepin (Sinequan) has been shown to be clearly superior to placebo in the treatment of such patients in at least two studies.[5] In more recent work carried out by Goldberg's group, imipramine appears to be at least equal to doxepin in effectiveness in this patient population.[17] A study comparing doxepin to amitriptyline is now in process. Although doxepin has been widely heralded as having special virtues in mixed anxiety and depression, it is entirely possible that this action is shared by other tricyclic antidepressants. Currently, doxepin and amitriptyline are probably most widely used because of their early sedative and hypnotic properties. Phenelzine (Nardil), a monoamine oxidase (MAO) inhibitor, has been studied in patients with mixed anxiety and depression by Nies and is also more effective than placebo.[18]

Drug Efficacy in Panic Attacks and in Phobic Anxiety

A growing body of studies has appeared in the literature attesting to the fact that tricyclic antidepressants—imipramine is the one most widely studied—have a unique and specific effect in patients who are subject to recurrent, severe panic attacks. Such patients usually also have secondary phobias which severely limit their social and vocational activities. Such patients are often dependent and clinging and afraid of being left alone, of travelling, of going to stores, or of going into other situations where they fear they may become subject to destructive panic without any help at hand. Although benzodiazepines may be of some use in handling the acute manifestations of a single panic attack, these syndromes are generally not responsive to sedative-hypnotic antianxiety agents. The panic attacks themselves are often nearly totally suppressed by tricyclic antidepressants.[19] Although some patients require doses similar to those used in depressive illnesses, others prove very sensitive to these drugs and may require only 10 mg per day and develop side effects with higher dosages. The antidepressant drugs often do not ameliorate the chronic anticipatory anxiety or the free-floating anxiety from which these patients suffer between panic attacks. Psychotherapeutic encouragement to increase their activities and change their life-styles once the panic attacks are removed may well be helpful, and the effects of benzodiazepines on anticipatory anxiety might recommend them for relieving these presumably secondary anxiety symptoms.

Drug Efficacy in Other Anxiety-like Conditions

Patients whose anxiety reflects, in large part, anxious responses to peripheral autonomic symptoms of anxiety may well be helped by propranolol.[7] This use, however, has not been approved by the Food and Drug Administration in the United States, although this drug is widely used for this purpose in England and has been shown to be more effective than placebo in at least one major trial. Since propranolol is not a hypnotic agent, it will likely not relieve the insomnia often associated with chronic anxiety symptoms.[20] The dosages used are generally between 30 and 120 mg per day, given in three or four divided doses. Beta-adrenergic blocking drugs such as propranolol have been reported to occasionally exacerbate depression.

Some patients with unstable personalities, or in whom anxiety is associated with distractability, hyperactivity, or obsessional features, may sometimes respond to low doses of antipsychotic drugs. Patients with more typical chronic anxiety symptoms may sometimes unpredictably fail to respond to antianxiety drugs or antidepressant drugs and may be found to respond uniquely to antipsychotic agents. These drugs should be used with caution and only in patients who are clearly unresponsive to other agents, since tardive dyskinesia has been shown to occur in nonpsychotic patients who receive these drugs for periods of as short as nine months. This investigator has personally seen six patients in the last two years who developed tardive dyskinesia on exposure to a single antipsychotic drug. The drugs involved have been thioridazine, chlorpromazine, trifluoperazine, thiothixene, and fluphenazine, which implies that all classes of antipsychotic drugs are liable to produce this highly undesirable effect.[21]

BEHAVIORAL TOXICITY

All the sedative-hypnotic drugs, including the benzodiazepines and to a lesser extent the tricyclic antidepressants, are liable to produce excessive sedation, drowsiness, and at higher doses, ataxia and drunken behavior. For this reason, patients receiving these drugs for the first time should be warned about the possible side effects, which may be incompatible with safe operation of motor vehicles or complicated machinery. Detailed psychologic testing of patients taking drugs of this class show that these agents have a disturbing tendency to effect errors of commission rather than errors of omission, and there may be settings in which errors of commission—doing the wrong thing, either impulsively or inadvertently—may have serious consequences. Since these drugs' sedative effects are strongest shortly after administration, and since their antianxiety effects may be longer lasting, giving them at bedtime rather than three times a day may help to minimize adverse effects issuing from excessive sedation.

These drugs are also disinhibiting agents. In one limited study, patients on chlordiazepoxide reported episodes of confrontation with spouse or boss which they felt to be good and positive; the boss or spouse may not have so judged these confrontations.[5] Essentially no serious work has been done on the real impact of antianxiety drugs on other individuals in the patient's environment. DiMascio's group has reported that benzodiazepines (diazepam to the greatest extent, and oxazepam to the least) have a tendency to elicit hostile, irritable behavior in relatively nonanxious volunteer subjects.[22] On the basis of his extensive data, Rickels claims that this phenomenon is not frequently observed in neurotic outpatient populations, but that nevertheless, it may be well for the treating clinician to keep a watchful eye on patients receiving these drugs.[12] The drugs have also occasionally been reported to be associated with increased depression and suicidal ideas—perhaps another example of their disinhibiting properties.[5]

The duration of the action of benzodiazepines may be both an asset and a liability. Diazepam and chlordiazepoxide are both relatively long lasting, with half-lives in the body of 24 hours or more. Oxazepam is shorter acting, with a half-life of perhaps 4 hours. Tybamate has the shortest half-life of all these drugs, a property which appears to be responsible for its inability to produce physical dependence in either man or dogs. It is worth noting in passing that Greenblatt has reported that both diazepam and chlordiazepoxide act less rapidly when given intramuscularly than when given orally.[23] Diazepam can, of course, be given intravenously for a rapid onset of action, but the clinical tendency to assume that intramuscular administration of drugs will produce the most rapid effect in emergency room situations is apparently incorrect for diazepam and chlordiazepoxide.

The autonomic-sedative drugs generally have anticholinergic properties which may cause side effects such as dry mouth, difficulty in urination, or, at very high doses or when given in combination with other drugs with anticholinergic properties, toxic delirium.

SAFETY

The benzodiazepines are probably among the safest drugs currently available for use in psychiatric patients in regard to overdose danger. It is almost impossible to commit suicide with benzodiazepines alone.[6][24] If they are taken in combination with other agents which depress the central nervous system, suicide is, of course, more likely. The barbiturates and the tricyclic antidepressants are both relatively dangerous in terms of suicide potential, with meprobamate occupying an intermediate status. The benzodiazepines are also free of the enzyme induction property common to barbiturates. When barbiturates are given, one must always worry that they are in fact speeding up the metabolism of other drugs given concomitantly, thereby making the other drug relatively less effective. The classic example is that of anticoagulant therapy: phenobarbital can, within two weeks, greatly accelerate the metabolism of anticoagulants. Conversely, when the phenobarbital is discontinued, the blood levels of anticoagulants will begin to rise within two weeks, perhaps to dangerous levels.[6]

ABUSE, MISUSE, AND INAPPROPRIATE USE

Given that antianxiety agents, particularly the benzodiazepines, are effective in the short-term treatment of anxiety—are they misused or abused? They are certainly very widely prescribed (80 million prescriptions in 1970), and a nationwide survey carried out in 1972 revealed that about 1 of every 7 adults in the United States had used an antianxiety drug at some time during the preceding year. About 1 in 20 had used antianxiety agents steadily for more than two months at some time during the preceding two years.[25] This use resembles that prevailing in western Europe.[26]

This data is vaguely reassuring, but it misses the point a bit. Until we know *when* antianxiety drugs should be used, it will be impossible to state whether any level of use constitutes over- or underuse. In the survey noted above, only one third of those respondents rating highest on dysphoria and stress had, in fact, used an antianxiety drug for their symptoms. On the other hand, many patients who come to psychiatrists for treatment give histories of prolonged use of benzodiazepines and are very resistant to having such drugs discontinued. Pharmacologically, it is clear that all the sedative-hypnotic antianxiety drugs can induce physical dependence.

At present, it is impossible to tell what proportion of psychiatric patients chronically treated with benzodiazepines is physically dependent, what proportion is only psychologically dependent, and what proportion requires these drugs for relief of chronic anxiety symptoms. Drug therapy is often expected, even demanded, by distressed patients. Hollister's suggestion of short-term two- to three-week courses of antianxiety drug therapy is well put and would help cut down on the number of patients who are chronically dependent on antianxiety drugs.[6] At the same time, it is unclear whether short-term psychotherapy is as effective as a benzodiazepine for anxiety symptoms. In busy primary care and clinic settings, drug therapy may well be the only feasible approach if brief supportive contacts are not sufficient.

REFERENCES

1. Shader, R.I. and Greenblatt, D.J.: The psychopharmacologic treatment of anxiety states. In Shader, R.I. (ed.): *Manual of Psychiatric Therapeutics.* Boston: Little, Brown & Co., 1975, pp. 27-38.

2. Chien, C.P., Stotsky, B.A. and Cole, J.O.: Psychiatric treatment for nursing home patients: drug, alcohol, and milieu. *Am. J. Psychiatry* 130: 5-12, 1972.

3. Cole, J.O. and Ryback, R.S.: Pharmacological therapy of alcoholism. In Tarter, R.E. and Sugerman, A.A. (eds.): *Alcoholism: Interdisciplinary Approaches to an Enduring Problem.* Reading, Mass: Addison-Wesley, 1976.

4. Harvey, S.C.: Hypnotics and sedatives. In Goodman, L.S. and Gilman, A. (eds): *The Pharmacological Basis of Therapeutics.* 5th ed. New York: MacMillan Publishing Co., 1975.

5. Cole, J.O. and Davis, J.M.: Antianxiety drugs. In Freedman, D.X. and Dyrud, J. (eds.): *American Handbook of Psychiatry.* Vol. 5. New York: Basic Books, 1975.

6. Hollister, L.E.: *Clinical Use of Psychotherapeutic Drugs.* Springfield, Ill: Charles C Thomas, 1973.

7. Lader, M. and Tyrer, P.J.: Response to propranolol and diazepam in somatic and psychic anxiety. *Br. Med. J.* 2:14-16, 1974.

8. Stein, L.S., Wise, C.D., and Berger, B.D.: Antianxiety action of benzodiazepines: decrease in activity of serotonin neurons in the punishment system. In Garattini, S., Mussini, E., and Randall, L.O. (eds.): *The Benzodiazepines.* New York: Raven Press, 1973, pp. 299-308.

9. Cook, L. and Sepinwall, J.: Behavior analysis of the effects and mechanisms of action of benzodiazepines. In Costa, E. and Greengard, P. (eds.): *The Mechanism of Action of Benzodiazepines.* New York: Raven Press, 1975.

10. Young, A.B., Zukin, S.R., and Snyder, S.H.: Interaction of benzodiazepines with central nervous system glycine receptors: possible mechanism of action. *Proc. Natl. Acad. Sci.* 71:2246-2250, 1974.

11. Irwin, S.: A rational framework for the development, evaluation, and use of psychoactive drugs. *Am. J. Psychiatry* 124 (suppl.):1-19, 1968.

12. Rickels, K.: Drug treatment of anxiety. In Jarvik, M.E. (ed.): *Psychopharmacology in the Practice of Medicine.* New York: Appleton-Century-Crofts, 1977, pp. 309-324.

13. McNair, D.M., Goldstein, A.P., Lorr, M. et al: Some effects of chlordiazepoxide and meprobamate with psychiatric outpatients. *Psychopharmacologia* 7:256-265, 1965.

14. Rickels, K., Hesbacher, P.T., Weise, C.T. et al: Pills and improvement, a study of placebo response in psychoneurotic outpatients. *Psychopharmacologia* 16:318-326, 1970.

15. Wheatley, D.: *Psychopharmacology in Family Practice.* London: William Heinemann Medical Books Ltd., 1973.

16. Derogatis, L.R., Lipman, R., Rickels, K. et al: The Hopkins Symptom Checklist (HSCL): a self-report symptom inventory. *Behav. Sci.* 19:1-15, 1974.

17. Goldberg, H.L., Finnerty, R.J., and Cole, J.O.: The effect of doxepin in the aged: interim report on memory changes and electrocardiographic findings. In Mendels, J. (ed.): *Sinequan (Doxepin HCL): A Monograph of Recent Clinical Studies.* New York: Excerpta Medica, 1975, pp. 65-69.

18. Ravaris, C., Nies, A. et al: A controlled study of multiple-dose phenelzine in depression-anxiety states. *Arch. Gen. Psychiatry* 33:347-352, 1976.

19. Klein, D.F.: Delineation of two drug-responsive anxiety syndromes. *Psychopharmacologia* 5:397-408, 1964.

20. Wheatley, D.: Comparative effects of propranolol and chlordiazepoxide in anxiety states. *Arch. Gen. Psychiatry* 115:1411-1412, 1969.

21. Gardos, G. and Cole, J.O.: Psychopharmacology update: tardive dyskinesia. *McLean Hosp. J.* 1:155-165, 1976.

22. DiMascio, A.: The effects of benzodiazepines on aggression: reduced or increased? *Psychopharmacologia* 30:95-102, 1973.

23. Greenblatt, D.J. and Shader, R.I.: *Benzodiazepines in Clinical Practice.* New York: Raven Press, 1974.

24. Greenblatt, D.J. and Shader, R.I.: Psychotropic drug overdosage. In Shader, R.I. (ed.): *Manual of Psychiatric Therapeutics.* Boston: Little, Brown & Co., 1975.

25. Perry, H.J., Balter, M.D., Meelinger, G.D. et al: National patterns of psychotherapeutic drug use. *Arch. Gen. Psychiatry* 28:769-783, 1973.

26. Balter, M., Levine, J., and Manheimer, D.: Cross-national study of the extent of anxiety/sedative drug use. *N. Engl. J. Med.* 290:769-774, 1974.

3 Drug Therapy of Insomnia
David J. Greenblatt, M.D.

Hypnotic drugs are extensively utilized by adults in the Western world. Surveys of psychotropic drug use among American adults indicate that approximately 4% of healthy, ambulatory Americans ingest hypnotic drugs on a regular basis.[1] Among hospitalized medical patients monitored by the Boston Collaborative Drug Surveillance Program, more than 80% are prescribed hypnotic drugs for the treatment of insomnia.[2] As there is such widespread use of hypnotic drugs, all health care professionals should be familiar with the clinical syndrome of insomnia and should understand the pharmacologic properties of hypnotic drugs as well as principles of the rational drug therapy of sleep disorders. This chapter briefly reviews such principles.

WHAT IS INSOMNIA?

Insomnia is a general term used by individuals who feel that they do not sleep the way they should or the way they would like to.[3] [4] The

The author is grateful for the collaboration of Drs. Richard I. Shader, Jan Koch-Weser, and Russell R. Miller and for the editorial assistance of Ann Werner.

Table 1
Subjective Reports and Objective Signs
Associated with Insomnia

Subjective Reports	Objective Signs
Takes too long to get to sleep	Long sleep latency
Wakes up too many times during the night	Many nocturnal awakenings
Nightmares or vivid dreams	Excessive rapid eye movement (REM) activity
Does not sleep long enough	Short sleep duration
Wakes up early in the morning and cannot get back to sleep	Early morning awakening
Feels groggy and "hung over" in the morning	Residual impairment of psychomotor function Residual EEG effects

subjective syndrome does not necessarily have specific objective correlates, but patients who complain of insomnia usually can point to one or more particular ways in which their sleep is disordered (Table 1). Many patients with insomnia will have a combination of subjective complaints, such as difficulty falling asleep, together with an excessive number of nocturnal awakenings. An individual's perception of whether or not his sleep is disordered depends upon his own particular needs and expectations. Some patients who fall asleep within three minutes of going to bed and who sleep for 10 hours may complain of insomnia; others who take a full hour to get to sleep and who sleep only 4 or 5 hours a night may consider their sleep to be perfectly normal. It is not uncommon for elderly individuals to complain of insomnia. Geriatric patients often tell physicians that they do not sleep the way they used to. In fact, a decreased need for sleep is a physiologic concomitant of aging and is not necessarily pathologic. It is often sufficient for physicians or health care professionals simply to reassure their elderly patients who complain of insomnia that a decreased need for sleep is a normal part of aging.

Insomnia often is not a primary disorder but rather a consequence of some underlying medical or psychiatric disease (Table 2). Physicians who choose to administer hypnotic drugs to patients with insomnia should carefully evaluate these individuals to determine whether such diseases are present. It would be quite irrational, for example, to prescribe a hypnotic drug to a patient with obstructive pulmonary disease whose nighttime restlessness or inability to sleep

Table 2
Diseases or Syndromes Which Can Cause Insomnia

Hypoxia
Hypoglycemia
Pulmonary congestion
Pain
Polyuria
Paroxysmal arrhythmias
Cerebral atherosclerosis
Thyrotoxicosis
Pheochromocytoma
Withdrawal from drugs (sedatives, alcohol, opiates, etc)
Use of other drugs (caffeine, amphetamines)
Anxiety
Depression

was due to hypoxia. Administration of a central depressant drug to such a patient may actually be contraindicated. Whenever an underlying disorder is responsible for clinical insomnia, therapy should be directed toward this underlying disease. Administration of hypnotics constitutes only symptomatic treatment, and may in fact do harm.

WHEN CAN HYPNOTIC DRUGS BE USED TO TREAT INSOMNIA?

Hypnotic drug therapy is rational when the sleep disorder is caused by short-term emotional stress or acute situational anxiety. This is often the case among hospitalized medical and surgical patients. Such individuals are exposed to an alien setting with its inevitable noise and disruption. They also experience the emotional stress associated with the presence or possibility of serious organic disease, and the disquieting anticipation of potentially uncomfortable diagnostic procedures. Assuming that disorders such as those in Table 2 have been ruled out, it is usually reasonable to provide symptomatic relief by prescription of hypnotic drugs. The physician and medical staff have control of the choice of drug, the frequency of administration, and its dosage. Hypnotic drug administration in hospitals rarely leads to untoward consequences such as dependence or overdosage. On the other hand, administration of hypnotic agents to ambulatory patients carries a considerably greater potential hazard and should be undertaken with caution.[5] The physician no longer has control of the dosage and the frequency of administration. It is essential that prescriptions for outpatients contain small numbers of pills and be nonrefillable. The patient should return for frequent follow-up evaluation of the sleep disorder. Like any other symptom, prolonged unexplained insomnia should not go without explanation and requires thorough medical and psychiatric evaluation.

EFFECTIVENESS OF HYPNOTIC DRUGS

A large number of hypnotic drugs are available by prescription in the United States (Table 3). Such drugs are forcefully promoted by the pharmaceutical industry. Extensive, controlled evaluation of these drugs has been carried out in a variety of patient populations, including ambulatory individuals with insomnia and geriatric populations who are institutionalized in nursing homes.[6] The results consistently demonstrate that all prescription hypnotic drugs available in the United States are more effective than placebo in the short-term treatment of insomnia. The drugs effectively reduce sleep latency, prolong the duration of sleep, reduce the number of nocturnal awakenings, improve the quality of sleep, and lead the patient to awaken feeling well rested. The choice of dosage is important. Clinical effectiveness can be consistently demonstrated only when adequate doses of the drugs are given. Apparent failures of therapy observed in clinical practice may be due not to any particular property of the drug, but rather

Table 3
Commonly Used Hypnotic Drugs

Generic Name	Trade Name
Barbiturates	
Secobarbital	Seconal
Pentobarbital	Nembutal
Amobarbital	Amytal
Butabarbital	Butisol
Phenobarbital	Luminal
Secobarbital plus amobarbital	Tuinal
Piperidinediones	
Glutethimide	Doriden
Methyprylon	Noludar
Chloral Derivatives	
Chloral hydrate	Noctec, Somnos
Chloral betaine	Beta-Chlor
Trichloroethyl phosphate (triclofos)	Triclos
Dichloralphenazone*	Welldorm
Benzodiazepines	
Flurazepam	Dalmane
Nitrazepam*	Mogadon
Lorazepam*	Ativan
Antihistamines	
Diphenhydramine	Benadryl
Hydroxyzine	Atarax, Vistaril
Quinazolines	
Methaqualone	Quaalude, Sopor
Methaqualone plus diphenhydramine*	Mandrax
Aliphatic Alcohols	
Ethchlorvynol	Placidyl

*Not currently available in the United States

to inadequate dosage. For example, clinicians commonly administer 500 mg of chloral hydrate, but controlled trials indicate that 500 mg is much less consistently effective than a dose of 1.0 g. Unless there is a compelling indication for using a low dose, it is usually reasonable to administer chloral hydrate in a dose of 1.0 g. Similar considerations apply to most other hypnotics.

When available hypnotic drugs are compared to each other in controlled studies using adequate dosages, the different drugs are usually found to be essentially indistinguishable. Again, all are more effective than placebo and are approximately equally effective in improving the subjective quality of sleep and the measurable sleep parameters. Thus, on the basis of short-term efficacy alone, no particular hypnotic drug is clearly preferable to any other.

It also appears that clinically effective doses of hypnotic agents produce unwanted effects with approximately equal frequency.[2] The most common side effect is the syndrome of "hangover," which is a feeling of residual drowsiness or heavy-headedness observed the morning after the drug is taken. The exact frequency or incidence of hangover among hypnotic drug users is very difficult to estimate. It depends on the type of study population, the method of assessment, and the dose. In most studies the incidence of clinically symptomatic hangover is relatively low. On the other hand, the electro-encephalogram 12 hours after ingestion of any hypnotic drug reveals a residual drug effect in 100% of cases. Furthermore, measurable concentrations of the drug will be present in the blood 12 hours after the dose in 100% of cases. Thus, although only a small percentage of subjects will complain of symptomatic hangover, all of them have objective evidence of the drug's presence in the body and its effect on the brain. This has important implications for patients who must perform tasks requiring a high level of intellectual and/or motor performance, such as operating an automobile, on the next day. All patients who are prescribed hypnotic drugs should be warned that although they have no subjective feelings of morning hangover, they might well have a subtle degree of impairment of intellectual or psychomotor performance.

Because prescription hypnotic drugs are very similar in clinical efficacy and toxicity, physicians must use criteria other than these to choose among available hypnotic agents. Such criteria include drug cost, the potential for drug abuse and addiction, the hazards associated with drug overdosage, drug interactions, and the extent to which the drug interferes with the normal physiology of sleep. These criteria do reveal differences among hypnotic agents which can allow a clinician to make the most rational choice of drug.

Barbiturates

Derivatives of barbituric acid have long been used as sedative and hypnotic agents in clinical medicine. They are time-tested and clearly effective when rationally prescribed on a short-term basis. Pharmacology textbooks customarily divide barbiturates into categories of short-, intermediate-, and long-acting preparations. These divisions are not really valid and probably are clinically irrelevant. None of the barbiturates commonly employed as hypnotic agents are truly short acting. Although secobarbital and pentobarbital have relatively rapid absorption rates and reach the systemic circulation rapidly when taken orally on an empty stomach, even these so-called short-acting preparations have low rates of clearance and fairly long elimination half-lives.[7] Thus, 24 hours after a single dose, relatively high drug concentrations remain in the blood. Furthermore, there is clear evidence of drug accumulation during chronic therapy.

The only potential advantage of hypnotic therapy with barbiturate derivatives is low cost. Many barbiturates are available by generic name and should be less expensive to the patient. In practice, however, this is seldom the case, because pharmacists rarely pass on the savings to consumers. For example, if secobarbital is prescribed by generic name and dispensed as an inexpensive generic brand, the cost to the patient should be relatively low. However, pharmacists will usually dispense such prescriptions using an expensive brand name such as Seconal because prescribing fees tend to be a percentage of wholesale drug cost rather than a fixed mark-up. Thus there is little incentive for most pharmacists to dispense inexpensive generic brands even when prescriptions are written as such. The potential financial savings associated with barbiturate therapy is seldom actually realized.

The list of disadvantages associated with barbiturate treatment of insomnia is long.[6] [8] Barbiturates are readily abusable drugs and commonly make their way into illicit street use. Doses of short-acting barbiturates only six to eight times larger than the usual therapeutic dosage, taken for a period of one to two months, will produce true physiologic addiction, in which an objective withdrawal syndrome follows abrupt discontinuation of the drugs. It is also well understood and widely observed that acute overdosage with barbiturates, particularly the so-called short-acting derivatives, produces a poisoning syndrome which is often serious and sometimes fatal. Furthermore, the margin of safety with barbiturates is small. While 100 to 200 mg of secobarbital, for example, may constitute an appropriate hypnotic dose, only 10 to 20 times as much may produce deep coma and possibly death.

Clinically important drug interactions can also occur during barbiturate therapy. Chronic administration of therapeutic doses of barbiturates to humans results in stimulation of hepatic microsomal enzymes.[6] [9] This can lead to increased clearance of certain other drugs, causing an apparent decrease in their clinical effectiveness. Clinically significant enzyme induction by barbiturates has been extensively documented in the case of oral anticoagulants. If a patient who has been taking a constant daily dose of an oral anticoagulant such as warfarin, and has thus achieved a stable prolongation of prothrombin time, is coadministered a barbiturate, the liver will metabolize the anticoagulant more rapidly and will therefore decrease its clinical effectiveness. In such patients, it may be necessary for the warfarin dosage to be increased in order to maintain its clinical efficacy. The real danger comes when barbiturate therapy is discontinued. If the dosage of anticoagulant is not appropriately reduced to account for the removal of the enzyme induction stimulus, excessive prolongation of the prothrombin time and bleeding reactions can occur. Although the potential clinical consequences of this interaction can be obviated by careful adjustment of anticoagulant dosage and close monitoring of prothrombin time, coadministration of barbiturates to anticoagulant-treated patients clearly adds a measure of uncertainty to their therapy.

Barbiturates interfere with the normal physiology of sleep.[3] [4] [6] Normal individuals spend about 25% of their total sleep time in the so-called rapid eye movement (REM), or dreaming, stage of sleep. When a barbiturate derivative is administered prior to sleep, the total amount of time spent in dreaming is greatly reduced. The consequences of this interference with REM sleep by barbiturates are not conclusively established. Many individuals take barbiturate hypnotics over a long period of time without any obvious clinical consequences. However, it does appear that long-term depression of dreaming by barbiturate hypnotics leads to a "dreaming debt," or increased pressure to dream. This dreaming debt may be responsible for the common clinical observation that barbiturate hypnotics tend to become ineffective when taken on a chronic basis.[10] [11] An individual may find that a 100-mg dose of secobarbital will improve his sleep during the first few nights of administration, but that it becomes ineffective when taken for a period of one to two weeks on a nightly basis. Such individuals often increase the dosage in order to restore the clinical effect of the drug. They may find that after one month of therapy they are taking 200 mg of secobarbital nightly, yet sleeping no better than they did prior to taking any medication. Furthermore, if the patient abruptly discontinues the barbiturate, a syndrome characterized by "REM rebound" may ensue, in which a supranormal percentage of sleeping time is spent in dreaming. Unfortunately, the rebound phenomenon is associated with nightmares, insomnia, and severely disordered sleep. It may be necessary for the patient to resume taking the drug if he is to get any sleep at all. This situation can be described as a state of hypnotic-drug dependence. It is not true addiction, but rather an unfortunate condition in which the patient is unable to sleep without medication because of the very unpleasant subjective manifestations of REM rebound. The interference of barbiturates with the normal physiology of sleep may be partly responsible for their decreasing effectiveness during chronic use, as well as for their ability to produce dependence.

Thus the disadvantages and hazards of barbiturate therapy of insomnia greatly outweigh the potential advantages. Again, the hazards are much greater for ambulatory individuals than for hospitalized patients. Although short-term administration of barbiturates under carefully controlled circumstances may be rational in some cases, it is generally wise for clinicians to avoid prescribing barbiturates for their patients with sleep disorders.[8]

Glutethimide and Methyprylon

These two agents are derivatives of the piperidinedione nucleus and are similar in structure and in pharmacologic activity.[6] Very little of a favorable nature can be said about them. Both are available by expensive trade names only and provide no potential financial savings. Both of these drugs interfere with REM sleep in much the same way as do barbiturates. Glutethimide is a potentially abusable drug. Furthermore, the poisoning syndrome associated with glutethimide overdosage can be very serious and is very difficult to treat because of the drug's high lipid-solubility and extensive binding to tissues. These two drugs therefore offer very little and need not be a part of any institution's formulary. Clinicians gain little or nothing by prescribing either of these two agents.

Chloral Derivatives

Chloral hydrate is among the very oldest of hypnotic agents. It is clinically effective, reasonably safe, and can be obtained as inexpensive generic brands. For reasons which are not established, serious poisoning with chloral hydrate is uncommonly observed, possibly because commercially available chloral hydrate capsules are very large and difficult to swallow in large numbers. Furthermore, most clinicians feel that chloral hydrate has the potential to produce gastric irritation. Thus, patients may vomit before large numbers of pills can be ingested. In any case, chloral hydrate appears to offer a considerable margin of safety over barbiturates and glutethimide.

Chloral derivatives do not cause clinically important microsomal enzyme induction in humans. However, this class of drugs can participate in other interesting, and sometimes important, drug interactions related to protein-binding displacement.[9] Trichloracetic acid, the final metabolite of all chloral derivatives, is tightly bound to human serum albumin. When chloral hydrate is coadministered with other agents which are tightly protein-bound, the generation of trichloracetic acid may lead to displacement of these other drugs from their binding sites on serum albumin. Since only the unbound fraction of such drugs is pharmacologically active, this may cause transient potentiation of their clinical effects. The interaction has been clearly demonstrated in the case of oral anticoagulants and may also be potentially important for drugs such as tolbutamide, diphenyl-hydantoin, furosemide, and possibly others.[12] Although the potentiation is transient, it is an interaction which should be considered when chloral derivatives are coadministered with other drugs having a high degree of protein binding.

Studies on the physiology of sleep following chloral administration are inconclusive. Most studies show that chloral derivatives do not interfere with the REM stage of sleep, although some studies show REM depression. It has also been observed that chloral derivatives, like barbiturates, tend to lose their effectiveness when given on a chronic basis. Further studies are needed to establish the rationale of long-term chloral hydrate therapy of insomnia.

In addition to chloral hydrate, at least two other chloral derivatives are available in the United States. These include chloral betaine and trichloroethyl phosphate (triclofos). Both of these drugs are clinically identical to chloral hydrate and are much more expensive. Another chloral derivative, available in Britain, is dichloralphenazone.

Benzodiazepines

The most familiar derivatives of the benzodiazepine nucleus available in the United States are chlordiazepoxide (Librium) and diazepam (Valium), but neither of these two drugs are promoted for the treatment of insomnia.[13] [14] In the United States, only flurazepam (Dalmane) is marketed and promoted specifically for the treatment of sleep disorders. However, it seems unlikely that flurazepam has any unique hypnotic properties not shared by other benzodiazepines.

Unfortunately, flurazepam is an expensive hypnotic agent. Outside of this disadvantage, it has other properties which make it a clinically useful and safe hypnotic agent.[13-16] As with other benzodiazepine derivatives, flurazepam appears to have a wide margin of safety. Serious poisoning following overdosage is probably unusual. Flurazepam does not interfere with oral anticoagulant therapy and it has no clinically important enzyme-inducing properties. Furthermore, flurazepam does not cause protein-binding displacement. Although flurazepam probably does not allow completely physiologic sleep, it appears to interfere with REM sleep to a much smaller degree than do barbiturates or glutethimide. Furthermore, following chronic flurazepam therapy, REM rebound does not occur. This may explain why flurazepam remains effective during chronic use.[11]

Clinicians who prescribe flurazepam should understand its metabolic pattern in the human body. Flurazepam is very rapidly transformed following oral administration to a metabolic product called desalkylflurazepam. This metabolite has pharmacologic activity similar to that of the parent drug. During chronic therapy with flurazepam, the parent drug does not accumulate, but there is considerable accumulation of the pharmacologically active metabolite.[17] Although no clinical consequences of the phenomenon have been clearly established, clinicians should be aware that there is a potential for cumulative effects of flurazepam during chronic therapy. Similar considerations apply to essentially all other hypnotic drugs, since accumulation of the parent compounds, their active metabolites, or both are possible during chronic administration.

Other benzodiazepine hypnotic agents may become available for clinical use in the near future. Nitrazepam (Mogadon) is widely used as a hypnotic in Britain and Europe and may eventually become available in the United States. Lorazepam (Ativan) is being extensively tested as a hypnotic and antianxiety agent. Other hypnotic benzodiazepines in the late stages of clinical testing include flunitrazepam and triazolam.

Antihistamines

Because of their nonspecific sedative effects, certain antihistamine derivatives are commonly used as hypnotics.[18] The most familiar of these are diphenhydramine (Benadryl) and hydroxyzine (Vistaril, Atarax). Although apparently effective in the treatment of insomnia, they are expensive drugs and have few advantages. It is commonly taught that antihistamines are somehow "milder" hypnotics and, as such, may be safe for elderly individuals and those with hepatic or renal disease. These myths are incorrect. Like other hypnotics, antihistamines are metabolized by the liver and are as unsafe as any other hypnotic drug in patients with hepatic insufficiency.[19] There is no evidence that antihistamines are safer than other hypnotics for elderly individuals. Because of their anticholinergic effects, they may actually be hazardous to the elderly, since such patients are prone to atropine-like manifestations of toxicity even with therapeutic doses. Furthermore, it is often observed that overdosage with antihistamines produces not central nervous system depression, but an acute agitated delirium resembling atropine poisoning. Thus, antihistamines are not particularly beneficial or useful hypnotic agents.

Miscellaneous Drugs

Methaqualone (Quaalude) is a quinazoline derivative which is used quite extensively as a hypnotic. It is sold by at least four different pharmaceutical manufacturing firms, each of which has provided its own expensive brand name. Methaqualone shares most of the potential hazards and disadvantages of the barbiturates. In addition, many individuals observe a type of peripheral paresthesia, termed a "buzz," which they may find pleasurable. This may account for the recent trend of methaqualone abuse, which has reached nearly epidemic proportions in some parts of the country.[20] Another hypnotic agent is ethchlorvynol (Placidyl), an acetylinic alcohol derivative. Although very little information is available about this drug, it appears to have no particular benefits as a hypnotic.

OVER-THE-COUNTER HYPNOTICS

A large number of alleged sleeping medications are available without prescription in supermarkets and drugstores.[21][22] Most of these contain an antihistamine such as methapyrilene, and/or scopolamine, an anticholinergic agent similar to atropine. Both of these compounds have very mild sedative properties. The preparations are sold under names such as Sominex, Nytol, Sleep-eze, Quiet World, Mr. Sleep, and many others. There is much concern, and with good reason, among legislators and regulatory agencies as to the efficacy of these preparations, and as to whether the extensive advertising claims made by their manufacturers are reliable. Controlled clinical trials of proprietary hypnotics suggest that they are no more effective than placebo and are considerably less effective than appropriate doses of prescription hypnotic agents.[21] Furthermore, they carry hazards of anticholinergic toxicity and have produced acute toxic delirium when taken in excessive quantities. They are also used by drug abusers as fully legal and easily available hallucinogens. No rationale exists for the clinical use of over-the-counter hypnotic products, and whenever possible patients should be discouraged from taking such agents.

CONCLUSION

Insomnia is a complex medical and psychiatric syndrome. It can be caused by or associated with a variety of other diseases. Non-investigative, symptomatic therapy of insomnia with hypnotic agents can never be considered rational. Sleep disorders should be thoroughly evaluated and treated only with full understanding of the potential benefits and hazards of hypnotic drug therapy.

REFERENCES

1. Greenblatt, D.J., Shader, R.I., and Koch-Weser, J.: Psychotropic drug use in the Boston area: a report from the Boston Collaborative Drug Surveillance Program. *Arch. Gen. Psychiatry* 32:518-521, 1975.

2. Miller, R.R. and Greenblatt, D.J. (eds.): *Drug Effects in Hospitalized Patients: Experiences of the Boston Collaborative Drug Surveillance Program, 1966-1975.* New York: John Wiley & Sons, Inc., 1976.

3. Greenblatt, D.J. and Miller, R.R.: Rational use of psychotropic drugs. I. Hypnotics. *Am.J. Hosp. Pharm.* 31:889-891, 1974.

4. Kales, A. and Kales, J.D.: Sleep disorders. *N. Engl. J. Med.* 290:487-499, 1974.

5. Clift, A.D.: Factors leading to dependence on hypnotic drugs. *Br. Med. J.* 3:614-617, 1972.

6. Greenblatt, D.J. and Shader, R.I.: The clinical choice of sedative-hypnotics. *Ann. Intern. Med.* 77:91-100, 1972.

7. Smith, R.B., Dittert, L.W., Griffen, W.O. et al: Pharmacokinetics of pentobarbital after intravenous and oral administration. *J. Pharmacokin. Biopharm.* 1:5-16, 1973.

8. Koch-Weser, J. and Greenblatt, D.J.: The archaic barbiturate hypnotics. *N. Engl. J. Med.* 291:790-791, 1974.

9. Koch-Weser, J. and Sellers, E.M.: Drug interactions with coumarin anticoagulants. *N. Engl. J. Med.* 285:487-498, 547-558, 1971.

10. Kales, A., Bixler, E.O., Tan, T.L. et al: Chronic hypnotic-drug use: ineffectiveness, drug-withdrawal insomnia, and dependence. *JAMA.* 227:513-517, 1974.

11. Kales, A., Kales, J.D., Bixler, E.O. et al: Effectiveness of hypnotic drugs with prolonged use: flurazepam and pentobarbital. *Clin. Pharmacol. Ther.* 18:356-363, 1975.

12. Sellers, E.M. and Koch-Weser, J.: Potentiation of warfarin-induced hypoprothrombinemia by chloral hydrate. *N. Engl. J. Med.* 283:827-831, 1970.

13. Greenblatt, D.J. and Shader, R.I.: *Benzodiazepines in Clinical Practice.* New York: Raven Press, 1974.

14. Greenblatt, D.J. and Shader, R.I.: Benzodiazepines. *N. Engl. J. Med.* 291:1011-1014, 1239-1242, 1974.

15. Greenblatt, D.J., Shader, R.I. and Koch-Weser, J.: Flurazepam hydrochloride. *Clin. Pharmacol. Ther.* 17:1-14, 1975.

16. Greenblatt, D.J., Shader, R.I. and Koch-Weser, J.: Flurazepam hydrochloride, a benzodiazepine hypnotic. *Ann. Intern. Med.* 83:237-241, 1975.

17. Kaplan, S.A., deSilva, J.A.F., Jack, M.L. et al: Blood level profile in man following chronic oral administration of flurazepam hydrochloride. *J. Pharm. Sci.* 62:1932-1935, 1973.

18. Tempero, K.F. and Hunninghake, D.B.: Antihistamines. *Postgrad. Med.* 48:149-155, August 1970.

19. Greenblatt, D.J., Shader, R.I. and Lofgren, S.: Rational psychopharmacology for patients with medical diseases. *Ann. Rev. Med.* 27:407-420, 1976.

20. Pascarelli, E.F.: Methaqualone abuse, the quiet epidemic. *JAMA.* 224:1512-1514, 1973.

21. Greenblatt, D.J. and Shader, R.I.: Non-prescription psychotropic drugs. In Jarvik, M.E. (ed.): *Psychotherapeutic Drugs in the Practice of Medicine.* New York: Appleton-Century-Crofts, 1977.

22. Greenblatt, D.J. and Shader, R.I.: Drug therapy: anticholinergics. *N. Engl. J. Med.* 288:1215-1219, 1973.

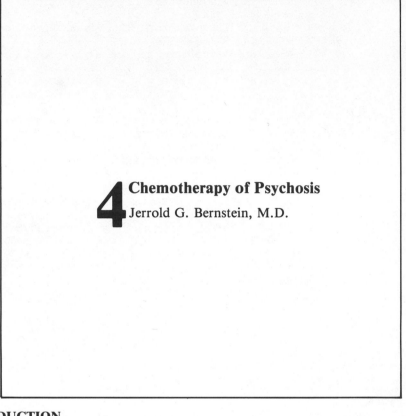

4 Chemotherapy of Psychosis

Jerrold G. Bernstein, M.D.

INTRODUCTION

In order for our patients to receive optimal benefits from chemotherapy, it is important that we have a clear understanding of the drugs available for clinical use, their mechanisms of action, and the techniques which will favor the desired therapeutic result and minimize unwanted drug side effects.

An understanding of currently available psychotropic drugs is facilitated by classifying them according to their primary therapeutic indication (Table 1). Trade names and generic drug names are used in the table, though generic names will generally be employed in this chapter. The term "major tranquilizer" has been widely used to describe the antipsychotic drugs. The latter term is preferable because it makes a clear statement about the nature of the effects that may be obtained with these drugs and avoids the confusion which may be associated with the word "tranquilizer," especially since the term "minor tranquilizer" has been used to describe the group of sedative-type agents, better known as antianxiety drugs.[1] It is very important to realize that the

40

pharmacology and mechanisms of action of the antipsychotic drugs are totally different from those of the antianxiety drugs.[1] This difference is more clearly expressed when the functional terms, rather than the terms major and minor tranquilizers, are employed. The antipsychotic drugs are unique in that they are capable of eliminating many of the prominent clinical signs and symptoms of psychosis, such as hallucinations, delusions, disordered thinking, and inappropriate behavior.[1][2] Often the desired therapeutic effect can be achieved with doses of antipsychotic drugs that produce minimal sedation or tranquilization. On the other hand, even in large doses, the antianxiety-type drugs have no beneficial effects against hallucinations, delusions, or disordered thinking, and they may produce profound sedation if the dose is increased in an attempt to achieve these benefits in a psychotic patient.[3] So indeed, there is something very unique about

Table 1
Classification of Psychotropic Drugs

Type of Drug	Generic Name	Trade Name
Antianxiety drugs		
Benzodiazepines	Chlordiazepoxide	Librium
	Diazepam	Valium
	Clorazepate	Taractan
	Oxazepam	Serax
Propanediol carbamate	Meprobamate	Equanil
Barbiturate	Phenobarbital	Luminal
Ethyl alcohol		
Antihistamine	Hydroxyzine	Atarax
Beta-adrenergic antagonist	Propranolol	Inderal
Antipsychotic drugs		
Aliphatic phenothiazine	Chlorpromazine	Thorazine
Piperidine phenothiazine	Thioridazine	Mellaril
Piperazine phenothiazines	Trifluoperazine	Stelazine
	Fluphenazine	Prolixin
	Perphenazine	Trilafon
Aliphatic thioxanthene	Chlorprothixene	Taractan
Piperazine thioxanthene	Thiothixene	Navane
Butyrophenone	Haloperidol	Haldol
Dihydroindolone	Molindone	Moban
Dibenzoxazepine	Loxapine	Loxitane
Antidepressant drugs		
Tricyclics	Amitriptyline	Elavil
	Imipramine	Tofranil
	Doxepin	Sinequan
MAO inhibitors	Phenelzine	Nardil
	Tranylcypromine	Parnate
	Pargyline	Eutonyl
CNS stimulants	Dextroamphetamine	Dexedrine
	Methylphenidate	Ritalin
Mood-stabilizing drug	Lithium carbonate	

the pharmacology of the compounds we call antipsychotic drugs. We are just beginning to recognize and understand this pharmacology, whose investigation is closely linked with our nascent understanding of the mechanism of psychotic illness.[4-6]

BIOCHEMICAL AND PHARMACOLOGIC ASPECTS OF PSYCHOSIS

It is important to review briefly some of the biochemical and pharmacologic knowledge relevant to the psychoses in order to understand more fully how the drugs under consideration bring about their ameliorative effects. A variety of investigations over the last quarter-century have pointed the way toward the recognition of biochemical abnormalities as a factor in the etiology and pathogenesis of the psychoses, particularly in schizophrenia and manic-depressive illness.[1 4 6 7] Numerous studies have implicated a variety of chemical substances derived from naturally occurring biogenic amines. Abnormal metabolites of biogenic amines, including norepinephrine, serotonin, acetylcholine, and histamine, have been found in the blood or urine of schizophrenic patients by a variety of researchers;[1 4 7] unfortunately, these studies have not always been replicable. Nevertheless, other kinds of data support biogenic amines as having a role in the mechanism of psychosis. A variety of substances, commonly termed *hallucinogens*, can produce an acute psychotic state in normal volunteers; all the known hallucinogens bear a chemical resemblance to naturally occurring biogenic amines.[4] For example, mescaline is a catecholamine derivative, while LSD (lysergic acid diethylamide) contains the indole nucleus as found in the naturally occurring substance serotonin. There are some theories of psychosis that suggest that naturally occurring biogenic amines may be abnormally changed in the body to produce a hallucinogenic substance.[7] When administered in large quantities to psychotic patients in remission, amino acids such as methionine and tryptophan, which facilitate synthesis of biogenic amines, may exacerbate psychotic symptoms. Furthermore, monoamine oxidase (MAO) inhibiting drugs, which are often used clinically in the treatment of depression, may produce acute psychotic symptoms when administered to individuals with an underlying schizophrenic illness. The mechanism by which MAO inhibitors may precipitate psychosis is apparently related to the mechanism of their antidepressant effect, namely, increasing the availability of catecholamine substances such as norepinephrine in the brain.[1 4]

Among the best information to support biochemical and pharmacologic mechanisms of psychosis is the evidence that a variety of drugs produce striking improvements in acutely psychotic patients.

Furthermore, it has become widely recognized that the antipsychotic effect of these drugs is dependent on their ability to decrease the availability or actions of certain neurotransmitters in the brain.[1][4][6] One of the earliest drugs shown to benefit acutely psychotic patients was reserpine, whose mechanism of action involves its ability to deplete or remove substances such as norepinephrine and serotonin from the brain.[1] All of the currently used effective antipsychotic drugs are capable of blocking dopamine receptors in the brain.[6] Despite the fact that there is a diversity in the chemical structure of the five groups of antipsychotic drugs (as shown in Table 1), each of these compounds exerts dopamine-blocking activity.[6] Furthermore, there is a parallel between the specificity of the various antipsychotic drugs for dopamine receptors and their ability to ameliorate clinical symptoms of the psychoses.[8] In addition to an apparent correlation between dopamine blockade and antipsychotic effects, it is also known that substances such as arecoline, with strong cholinergic actions, may temporarily alleviate psychotic symptoms in experimental situations, although the duration of action of this compound is too short to be of practical clinical usefulness.[1][5]

ANTIPSYCHOTIC CHEMOTHERAPY

Antipsychotic drugs are indicated in the acute treatment of psychoses, including schizophrenia, mania, and psychotic depression.[2] These drugs are also useful in long-term maintenance of schizophrenic patients and in the control of acute exacerbations in the condition of patients with chronic schizophrenia.[9] Antipsychotic drugs are frequently useful in helping to control the agitation, confusion, hallucinations, delusions, and disordered thinking associated with organic brain syndromes.[1][2] Those antipsychotic drugs with higher sedative potency may be useful in alleviating severe anxiety, especially when the anxiety has been of long duration or resistant to other pharmacologic agents.[2]

In order to achieve maximal benefits with antipsychotic drug treatment, it is necessary to have a clear view of the techniques and goals of antipsychotic chemotherapy as well as of the indications for these drugs. Indeed, once the proper drug is ordered for a given patient, an adequate therapeutic dose must be determined and the patient must take the medication as prescribed to achieve the desired response. Many apparent failures of drug treatment can be attributed to the use of inadequate dosage or to the refusal of the patient to take the prescribed medication regularly. One might apply a "bill of rights" for drug prescribing which includes four basic points. First, the right drug must be administered; that is, the characteristics of the compound prescribed must be capable of alleviating the symptoms of disease displayed by the patient. Second, the right dosage of medication must be employed. Therapeutic failures are most often related to inadequate dosage, but therapeutic misadventures may also be caused by adverse effects of excessive medication. The third point of this bill of rights is the need to administer the medication according to the schedule and route appropriate for the drug and the patient. Since most psychotropic drugs produce adequate therapeutic responses when administered in a single daily dose, this schedule is preferable from the standpoint of convenience to the patient and of a lesser likelihood of the patient forgetting to take the medication.[1] [2] In the initial phases of drug treatment, while the patient's response to the medication is being evaluated, divided daily doses generally need to be administered. Under most circumstances, antipsychotic drugs produce adequate absorption and favorable therapeutic response with oral administration.[1] In selected circumstances, acute administration of intramuscular preparations is necessary to provide control. A number of individuals tell us, by both their history and current behavior, that they are not going to take antipsychotic medication over a prolonged period. For such patients, periodic administration of the various long-acting antipsychotic compounds often achieves the desired therapeutic response.[2] Finally, perhaps one of the most important points in the bill of rights is that the patient has the right to be informed in some detail about the nature of the medication to be administered, the beneficial effects which may be achieved, and the unwanted side effects which he may experience. Improved dialogue between patient and prescribing physician can be expected to facilitate a favorable therapeutic response and to increase the likelihood of the patient's complying with the recommended medication regimen.

CHOOSING THE APPROPRIATE ANTIPSYCHOTIC DRUG

Having discussed the mechanism of action, techniques, and goals of antipsychotic chemotherapy, let us now explore some of these principles in relation to the application of specific drugs in the treatment of psychotic illness. We now have approximately 15 effective antipsychotic drugs at our disposal. The first such drug to become available for clinical use in the United States was chlorpromazine (Thorazine), introduced in 1954. Many reasons may be presented for the development of a large number of drug products in this field of therapeutics; perhaps the most important is that none of the available drugs is perfect and there is a continuing attempt to develop more effective drugs with fewer unwanted effects. Thus far, there is no product available in any area of therapeutics which is totally free of adverse effects. Currently available antipsychotic drugs may be divided into five groups, based upon differences in their chemical structures (Table 1). It is generally believed that all of these compounds exert their beneficial effect as a result of their ability to block dopamine receptors in the brain. Furthermore, these compounds all share a variety of unwanted effects which derive from common features in their pharmacology.[1] [2] The extent and relative severity of side effects among the different antipsychotic drugs vary considerably and may form a logical basis for choosing one agent over another for use in a given patient.

In order for these drugs to have gained approval for marketing, the manufacturers had to demonstrate the efficacy and relative safety of each of the compounds in question in clinical investigative studies. More extensive clinical experience with a drug improves the validity of our knowledge of the safety and efficacy of that particular agent. Although the effective dosage of a given compound varies considerably from patient to patient, the goal of treatment is always the greatest improvement of symptoms with the minimum of adverse effects.

Common Adverse Effects

Four of the most widely experienced adverse effects associated with antipsychotic drugs are: *sedation, hypotension, anticholinergic effects*, and *extrapyramidal effects (parkinsonian symptoms)*. In weighing the relative advantages and disadvantages of the antipsychotic drugs currently available for clinical use, it is worthwhile to consider them in relation to their individual likelihoods of producing each of these unwanted effects.

Chlorpromazine (Thorazine), chlorprothixene (Taractan), and thioridazine (Mellaril) exert the most pronounced sedative effects. Although sedation may be an advantage in the treatment of some agitated or belligerent patients, the primary goal of treatment with these drugs is to alleviate specific psychotic symptoms while leaving the patient alert and awake so that he can function, either on the ward in the hospital or, eventually, out in the community. The above-mentioned compounds tend to produce a high degree of sedation relative to their specific antipsychotic effects. At the other end of the spectrum, the piperazine phenothiazines such as trifluoperazine (Stelazine) and fluphenazine (Prolixin), and the piperazine thioxanthene derivative thiothixene (Navane), produce relatively minor sedative effects, which may be advantageous in more withdrawn or depressed patients. The butyrophenone haloperidol (Haldol) has relatively mild sedative effects at usual maintenance dosages. However, when desirable, a greater degree of sedation can be obtained in the agitated patient through the use of larger doses.

Two additional antipsychotic drugs have become available more recently; because of less extensive clinical experience with these drugs, our knowledge of them is somewhat limited. Loxapine (Loxitane) appears to be in an intermediate position with respect to sedative effects relative to antipsychotic action.[10] Molindone (Moban) appears to produce relatively little sedation, and some studies have attributed a slight stimulant action to this drug. The latter, however, is difficult to clarify and may well be a manifestation of akathisia produced by this compound.[10]

The clinical experience with molindone and loxapine has thus far failed to indicate any particular therapeutic advantage of these new drugs over other, already available antipsychotic agents—from the standpoint of either efficacy or side effects.[10] They also suffer the disadvantage of thus far being available for administration only by the oral route. Nevertheless, patients who have failed to respond to adequate dosages of available agents, or who have had intolerable side effects, may well benefit from a trial of one of these newer additions to the therapeutic armamentarium.

The hypotensive action of antipsychotic drugs is potentially dangerous, not only because of the primary effect upon the circulatory system, but also because of related secondary risks. Patients may develop considerable postural hypotension and may actually faint and sustain physical injury with some antipsychotic compounds.[1][2] This risk is particularly great in elderly patients, in those with underlying cardiovascular disease, and in those receiving other medications affecting the cardiovascular system.[14][15] The hypotensive action of antipsychotic drugs is based upon the ability of some of these compounds to exert pronounced alpha-adrenergic blockade with consequent peripheral vasodilation and a fall in both peripheral resistance and blood pressure. Chlorpromazine, chlorprothixene, and thioridazine are the most potent alpha-adrenergic blocking agents among the drugs under consideration, and therefore are most likely to produce hypotensive reactions of clinical significance. The hypotensive actions of piperazine phenothiazines such as trifluoperazine and fluphenazine and of the piperazine thioxanthene derivative thiothixene are considerably less than those of the previously mentioned drugs. Among the antipsychotic drugs, haloperidol has the least effect on the cardiovascular system.[1] [14] This drug has little likelihood of producing hypotension, even in relatively large doses, and does not produce the electrocardiographic changes which are frequently seen with phenothiazine compounds.[15] Hypotensive reactions have been associated with the use of both loxapine and molindone, although the degree of their hypotensive potential is difficult to establish at the present time in light of relatively limited clinical experience with both of these newer drugs.[10]

Among the antipsychotic agents, thioridazine possesses the most pronounced anticholinergic activity.[5] It is the most likely to induce blurred vision, dry mouth, constipation, urinary retention, decreased perspiration, and an increased heart rate. Chlorpromazine and chlorprothixene also possess relatively high degrees of anticholinergic potency, while trifluoperazine, fluphenazine, and haloperidol have less pronounced anticholinergic actions, and in usual therapeutic doses are somewhat less likely to induce the previously described symptoms of cholinergic blockade.[5] [14] Both molindone and loxapine are known to exert anticholinergic effects, though their relative potency in this regard must be determined by further clinical research.[10]

One interesting and potentially advantageous aspect of high anticholinergic potency among antipsychotic drugs is that those compounds with greater anticholinergic action tend to produce fewer extrapyramidal effects.[5] Indeed, among the available antipsychotic drugs, thioridazine appears least likely to produce severe parkinsonian reactions.[5] [14] As has previously been mentioned, there is a strong parallel between antipsychotic potency and dopamine receptor blocking activity among the antipsychotic drugs.[6] [8] Similarly, the likelihood of a given compound inducing unwanted extrapyramidal effects appears to parallel both its antipsychotic potency and its dopamine-blocking action.[4] In patients particularly susceptible to extrapyramidal reactions, thioridazine may be the drug of choice if psychotic symptoms can be controlled within the range of dosage considered safe: that is, less than 800 mg per day. The upper dosage limit must be followed with this particular drug because higher doses have been associated with irreversible retinal damage and visual impairment.[14] Chlorpromazine and chlorprothixene, which both possess rather strong anticholinergic actions associated with lower dopamine-blocking activity, are of intermediate potency in producing parkinsonian reactions.[1] [14] The more potent antipsychotic drugs, such as trifluoperazine, fluphenazine, thiothixene, and haloperidol, are more likely to induce extrapyramidal reactions.[14] Generally speaking, however, dosage adjustment or coadministration of antiparkinsonian drugs will alleviate or entirely prevent unwanted extrapyramidal reactions.[1] [14] One interesting aspect with haloperidol is that with higher doses, particularly those exceeding 60 mg per day, there is a progressive decline in the incidence and severity of extrapyramidal reactions. This seemingly paradoxical effect may be explained by the fact that the greater anticholinergic action associated with larger doses of haloperidol antagonizes the drug's extrapyramidal effects. Again, although experience with loxapine and molindone is limited, it appears that loxapine produces considerable extrapyramidal effects, perhaps comparable to the parkinsonian reactions incurred with piperazine phenothiazine compounds such as trifluoperazine. Molindone has also been associated with extrapyramidal reactions, though the relative severity and likelihood of these reactions is difficult to categorize on the basis of current clinical experience with this compound.[10]

PHASES OF ANTIPSYCHOTIC DRUG TREATMENT

Having compared the available antipsychotic drugs with respect to their unwanted effects, let us consider the initiation and course of antipsychotic chemotherapy as applied to schizophrenic patients. The drug treatment of psychosis may be divided into three phases. The initial phase of treatment in the schizophrenic or manic patient is aimed at the control of agitation, hallucinations, delusions, and disordered thinking. Since the mechanism by which these drugs achieve their desired effect is generally thought to be related to blockade of dopamine receptors in the brain, perhaps the initial goal of treatment should be to provide adequate dosage of medication to achieve suitable drug concentrations within the brain. The term *pharmacolysis of psychosis* might be used to describe the initial phase of drug treatment of an acutely psychotic patient. At this point medication is administered in gradually increasing dosages, adjusted according to the patient's response, in order to achieve improvement or control of symptoms.[10] [11]

Recalling some of the individual characteristics of the drugs discussed, one might well begin treatment with haloperidol, particularly in the more agitated psychotic patient. The usual initial dosage for a young to middle-aged, otherwise healthy individual is 5 mg four times daily. The patient is then observed carefully and his need for additional haloperidol, beyond the 5 mg four times daily, is assessed. If indicated, the dosage is gradually increased as required, with additional haloperidol given in 5- to 10-mg increments at hourly intervals, if necessary, to control anxiety, agitation, or other disturbing symptoms. Depending upon the patient's clinical response, behavior, and side effects, the dosage may then be adjusted either downward or (more commonly) upward to achieve the desired effect. Most often, a dosage of 20 to 60 mg of haloperidol daily is appropriate in the initial phase of treatment. Sometimes, however, the daily dosage needs to be increased still further—to 100 mg or occasionally more—during the first week or two of treatment. If adequate dosages are employed, psychotic symptoms will be seen to diminish within the first few days of chemotherapy, and at the same time, the patient will remain alert and be able to participate in psychotherapeutic aspects of the hospital program.

The second phase of treatment with antipsychotic drugs may be called the *stabilization phase*, wherein the dosage of antipsychotic medication is gradually reduced, generally during the second to fourth week of treatment, the goal being to maintain control of symptoms and minimize unwanted drug side effects in the schizophrenic patient. In acutely manic patients, lithium carbonate is generally started in the early phase of treatment and its dosage adjusted to achieve adequate blood levels of the drug as the antipsychotic agent is gradually withdrawn.[12][13] Generally, the dosage of antipsychotic agent can be stabilized at about one half of the maximal dosage previously required.

The third phase of antipsychotic drug treatment of the schizophrenic patient may be termed the *maintenance phase*. In this stage the dosage of antipsychotic agent is gradually reduced to the lowest level necessary to achieve symptom control while minimizing side effects.[9] The maintenance dosage of haloperidol, generally in the range of 10 to 30 mg daily, may be achieved by the end of hospitalization without jeopardizing the clinical improvement which has been observed. Reappearance of psychotic symptoms during dosage reduction should be countered by a temporary increase in the dosage of medication. On the other hand, the persistence of unwanted side effects may be an indication that dosage reduction should be accomplished at a more rapid pace. During the maintenance phase of treatment with antipsychotic drugs, drug holidays may occasionally be employed. It is often desirable in long-term treatment to discontinue medication at some point in order to ascertain the continuing clinical need for antipsychotic medication and to minimize the risk of long-term treatment complications such as tardive dyskinesia.[9][10]

Extrapyramidal reactions which develop during the course of treatment with haloperidol or other antipsychotic drugs may be managed by the addition of an antiparkinsonian medication to the regimen. One to 2 mg of benztropine (Cogentin) or trihexyphenidyl (Artane) two to four times daily is generally effective in controlling unwanted extrapyramidal reactions. When treating patients with antipsychotic medications, one should be particularly watchful for the development of akathisia. This effect should not be confused with anxiety or activation and should be treated specifically with anti-parkinsonian medication. Although there are a variety of effective antiparkinsonian medications, all are generally associated with the production of blurred vision and dry mouth (among other anti-cholinergic symptoms), since their mechanism of action generally is related to cholinergic blockade. On the other hand, amantadine (Symmetrel) has been shown to be highly effective in controlling drug-induced extrapyramidal reactions.[15] This compound appears to exert its antiparkinsonian effect primarily through an action on dopamine receptors rather than by the more widespread anticholinergic action seen with other antiparkinsonian drugs.[16] Amantadine is generally an effective antiparkinsonian agent when administered in a dosage of 100 mg twice daily.

CONCLUSION

Lastly, one should keep in mind another important principle of rational pharmacotherapy. For optimal clinical response with minimal complications, it is generally preferable to avoid polypharmacy. There is rarely a need to use two or more antipsychotic drugs simultaneously in the treatment of any patient. It is far better to employ larger doses of a single agent, or to change to a different agent, if a satisfactory response has not been achieved after several weeks of adequate treatment than it is to pyramid one drug on top of another. Treatment with multiple antipsychotic drugs is less likely to facilitate the desired therapeutic response and more likely to induce the development of side effects and complications.

REFERENCES

1. Byck, R.: Drugs and the treatment of psychiatric disorders. In Goodman, L.S. and Gilman, A. (eds.): *The Pharmacological Basis of Therapeutics.* New York: MacMillan Publishing Co., 1975.

2. Hollister, L.E.: *Clinical Use of Psychotherapeutic Drugs.* Springfield, Ill: Charles C Thomas, 1973.

3. Greenblatt, D.J. and Shader, R.I.: *Benzodiazepines in Clinical Practice.* New York: Raven Press, 1974.

4. Snyder, S.H., Banerjee, S.P., Yamamura, H.I. et al: Drugs, neurotransmitters and schizophrenia. *Science* 184:1234-1253, 1974.

5. Snyder, S., Greenberg, D., and Yamamura, H.I.: Antischizophrenic drugs and brain cholinergic receptors. *Arch. Gen. Psychiatry* 31:58-61, 1974.

6. Snyder, S.H.: The dopamine hypothesis of schizophrenia: focus on the dopamine receptor. *Am. J. Psychiatry* 133:197-202, 1976.

7. Gillin, J.C., Kaplan, J., Stillman, R. et al: The psychedelic model of schizophrenia: the case of N,N-dimethyltryptamine. *Am. J. Psychiatry* 133:203-208, 1976.

8. Seeman, P. and Lee, T.: Antipsychotic drugs: direct correlation between clinical potency and presynaptic actions on dopamine neurons. *Science* 188:1217-1219, 1975.

9. Davis, J.M.: Overview: maintenance therapy in psychiatry: I. Schizophrenia. *Am. J. Psychiatry* 132:1237-1245, 1975.

10. Davis, J.M.: Recent developments in the drug treatment of schizophrenia. *Am. J. Psychiatry* 133:208-214, 1976.

11. Anderson, W.H., Kuehnle, J.C., and Catanzano, D.M.: Rapid treatment of acute psychosis. *Am. J. Psychiatry* 133:1076-1078, 1976.

12. Gershon, S. and Shopsin, B.: *Lithium: Its Role in Psychiatric Research and Treatment.* New York: Plenum Press, 1973.

13. Baldessarini, R.J. and Lipinski, J.F.: Lithium salts: 1970-1975. *Ann. Intern. Med.* 83:527-533, 1975.

14. Shader, R.I. and DiMascio, A.: *Psychotropic Drug Side Effects.* Baltimore: The Williams & Wilkins Co., 1970.

15. Fowler, N.O., McCall, D., Chou, T.C. et al: Electrocardiographic changes and cardiac arrhythmias in patients receiving psychotropic drugs. *Am. J. Cardiol.* 37:223-230, 1976.

16. Fann, W.E. and Lake, C.R.: Amantadine versus trihexyphenidyl in the treatment of neuroleptic-induced parkinsonism. *Am. J. Psychiatry* 133:940-943, 1976.

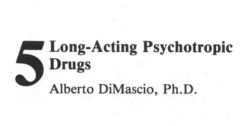

5 Long-Acting Psychotropic
Drugs

Alberto DiMascio, Ph.D.

ROLE OF LONG-ACTING ANTIPSYCHOTICS

Since the advent of psychotropic drugs in psychiatry 20 years ago, there have been a number of innovative milestones that have resulted in the more effective treatment of psychiatric patients and also in the production of fewer adverse reactions. Salient among these innovations has been the development of nonphenothiazine classes of neuroleptics: thioxanthenes (chlorprothixene and thiothixene), butyrophenones (haloperidol), diphenylbutylpiperidines (pimozide), dibenzodiazepines (loxapine), and the dihydroindole compound molindone. The development of these compounds has resulted in drugs with greater specificity and lessened toxicity.

None of these drugs are of value, however, if patients do not take them at the dosage that has been prescribed, or if their bodies do not absorb the orally administered drug effectively.[1] It has been estimated that 10% to 25% of schizophrenic inpatients somehow fail to ingest the prescribed dosage, and that 25% to 50% of schizophrenic outpatients deviate from or default on their medication regimens.[2] This

52

has obvious consequences in terms of the relapse rate and revolving door syndrome. Apart from the personal implications, drug defaulting and an increase in relapses involves an enormous economic waste. Representing a more bizarre consequence of this behavior was the report that a fatal epidemic among seagulls near a large mental hospital bordering the seacoast was due to their ingesting psychotropic drug tablets which had been discarded by the patients.

The development of long-acting formulations (both injectable and oral) carries the potential to remedy these two treatment liabilities. "Long-acting" as used here does not refer to drugs that can be given once a day (most of the psychotropic drugs now available can be so administered) but rather once a week or even less often. These new formulations have already made an impact on the treatment of the unreliable drug taker, the poor oral absorbers, and those patients being treated in outpatient settings who are too ill to assume responsibility for their own drug taking.

Among these extremely long-acting drugs are modifications of other antipsychotics: the piperazine-phenothiazine fluphenazine has been converted to fluphenazine enanthate and fluphenazine decanoate; the thioxanthene analogue of fluphenazine, to fluphenthixol decanoate; and the piperidine-phenothiazine pipothiazine, to pipothiazine undecylenate and pipothiazine palmitate. Two diphenylbutylpiperidines, fluspirilene and penfluridol, have also been developed. (See Figure 1.)

CHEMICAL ADAPTATIONS

Fluphenazine hydrochloride was converted into fluphenazine enanthate by first esterifying the side chain and combining it with heptanoic acid ester, thus producing a large, more complex molecule that has to be hydrolyzed by the body in order to release the free fluphenazine. To retard this hydrolysis, the molecule was prepared in a sesame oil vehicle that is used for intramuscular injection. This alteration resulted in an effective antipsychotic (fluphenazine enanthate) that required administration only every other week. The chemists next used decanoic acid as the esterifying agent since the greater number of carbons in the decanoic acid ester made the hydrolysis of the drug a slower process and resulted in a longer-acting and smoother-releasing formulation. Clinical experience has, indeed, shown that this drug (fluphenazine decanoate) can be given once every three weeks,[3] or even less often in many patients, for the effective treatment of schizophrenia (Figure 1A).

(A)

FLUPHENAZINE

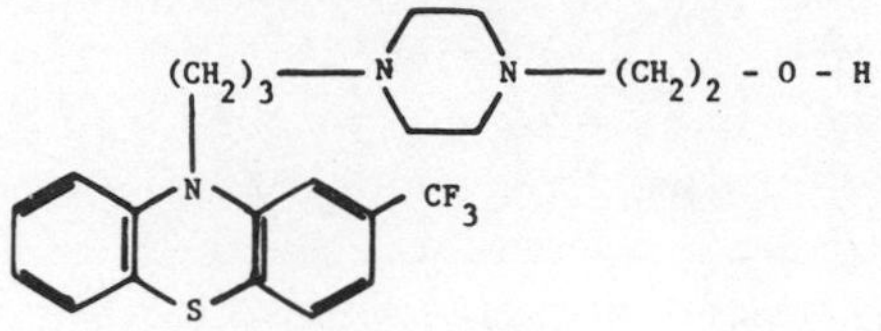

FLUPHENAZINE ENANTHATE

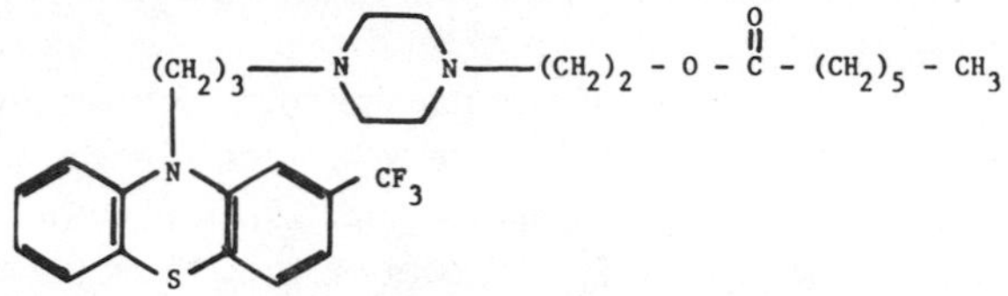

FLUPHENAZINE DECANOATE

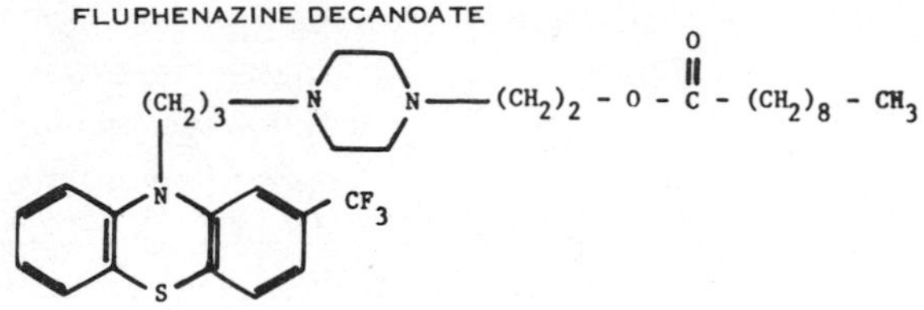

(B)

FLUPENTHIXOL DECANOATE

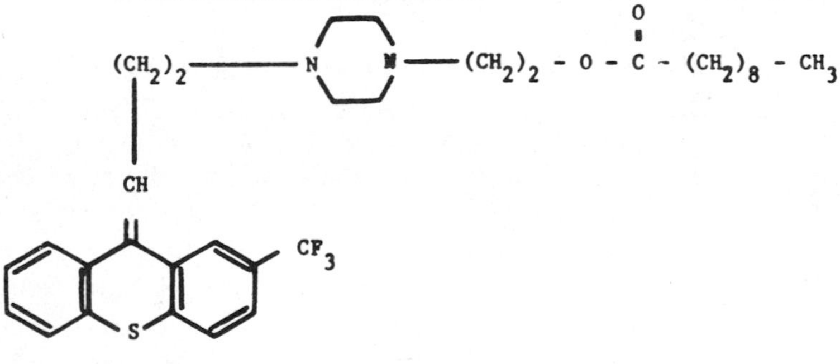

Figure 1, A—D. Chemical structures of long-acting antipsychotic drugs.

(C)

PIPOTHIAZINE UNDECYLENATE

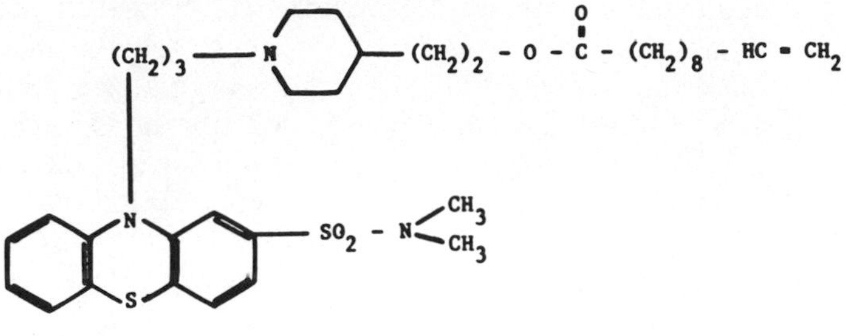

PIPOTHIAZINE PALMITATE

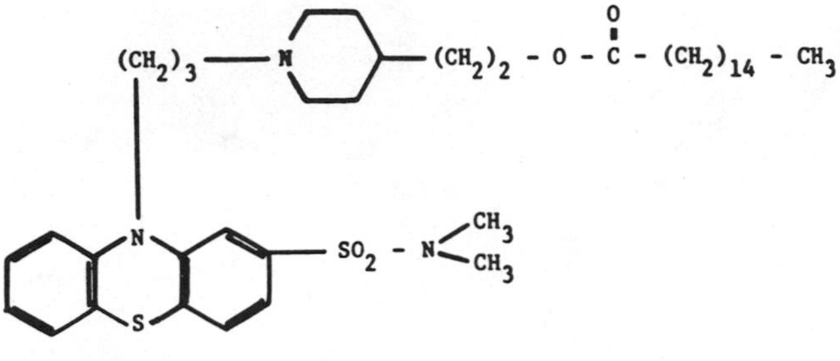

(D)

BENZPERIDOL

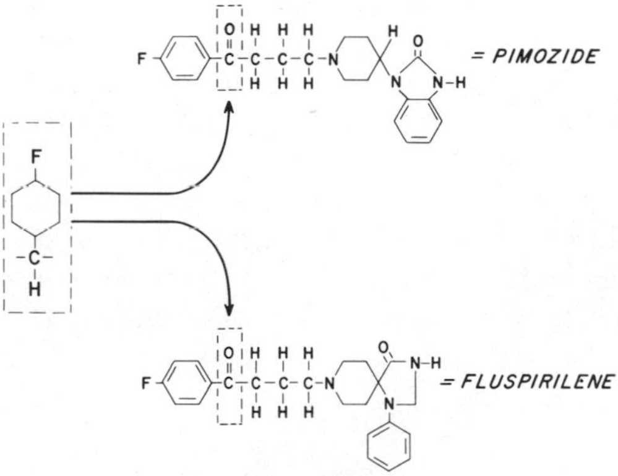

= PIMOZIDE

= FLUSPIRILENE

SPIROPERIDOL

PENFLURIDOL

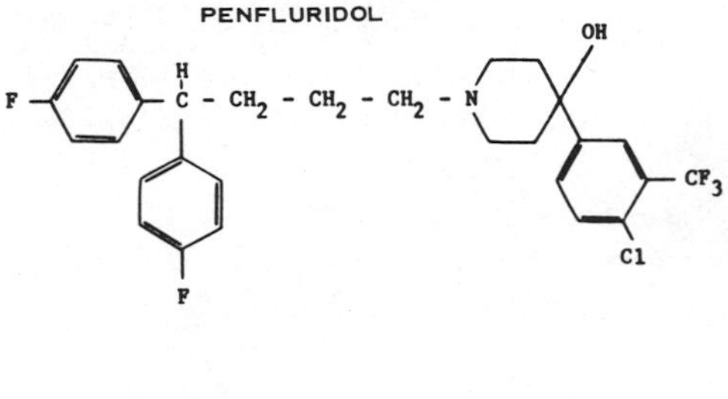

One of the reasons that fluphenazine and not other, earlier-marketed phenothiazines could be used was that fluphenazine is a low-dose, high-potency drug. It was possible to place all the free fluphenazine needed for a two- to four-week period in a small amount of a solution that could be injected comfortably. To deliver all the chlorpromazine, or even all the trifluoperazine, that would be needed for a two- or three-week period, one would have to inject a considerable amount of the carrying vehicle.

Researchers, witnessing the growth in the use of these two fluphenazine products, began seeking other drugs that could be similarly formulated. One approach was to convert the fluphenazine decanoate to the thioxanthene analogue by replacing the nitrogen in the phenothiazine nucleus with a double-bond carbon in the 10 position. This molecular manipulation resulted in a drug called flupenthixol decanoate, which is given once every other week (Figure 1B).[4] Other chemists modified a phenothiazine used in Europe, pipothiazine, which consists of a phenothiazine nucleus with a sulfonamide at the 2 position and a piperidine side chain at the 10 position. It is thus similar to thioproperazine (Majeptil) and to piperacetazine (Quide). This drug was esterified in two forms (undecylenate and palmitate), both of which are also dissolved in sesame oil: the undecylenate lasts two weeks, and the palmitate lasts four weeks (Figure 1C).[5]

Another chemical maneuver was to take a structurally different antipsychotic drug class, the butyrophenones, and develop a chemical class, diphenylbutylpiperidines, in which the carbonyl group in the propylene chain is replaced by a fluorophenyl group.[6] Depending on the aromatic substituent on the phenyl ring—or on replacement of the phenyl ring—three new, long-acting, effective antipsychotics could be produced: pimozide, fluspirilene, and penfluridol (Figure 1D). Only the latter two are effective for a week or more after a single dose; fluspirilene is injected and penfluridol is given orally.[7] [8]

EVALUATING THE LONG-ACTING PSYCHOTROPICS

What can be said about these drugs—as a group and individually? First, it is known that, except for penfluridol (the only oral form), when the drug is injected the patient will have the drug in his system. There is no way that he can cheek it, spit it out, or regurgitate it and thus retard his treatment and rehabilitation. The use of these drugs gives some feeling of security to the patient, the patient's family, his employer, and the hospital staff.

The incidence and frequency of side effects with the injectable long-acting drugs are not greater than with the oral, short-acting forms. In fact, there are some data showing that the former may produce even fewer side effects because of the lower dosages required for effective treatment. The fears once held that numerous patients would show untreatable and long-lasting extrapyramidal symptoms when administered the long-acting forms now appear to be groundless. There is no need, as some previous investigators have advocated, to place a patient on an oral dose of the medication prior to initiating the injectable form.

The required dosage of the injectable ester is often but a fraction of the amount of medication required with the oral form. Patients who may have required 40 mg daily of oral fluphenazine can be equally effectively maintained on a 25-mg injection of fluphenazine decanoate once every three weeks. Such a patient would require 840 mg of the oral drug, but only 25 mg of the injectable decanoate—about 3% of the oral dose—over this three-week period. Patients who require 1000 mg of chlorpromazine daily to control their psychotic states have been maintained on 50 mg of fluphenazine decanoate once every two weeks: 14,000 mg of the oral form vs 50 mg of the injectable (about 0.35% of the amount of oral medication). (See Table 1)

Just as with the oral forms, there is considerable variation among patients in the dosage required to obtain clinical benefit and in the duration of action of the injectable forms. Duration of activity varies from one to eight weeks with these formulations. These variations require that the physician carefully titrate dosage amounts and injection intervals to maximize clinical effectiveness and minimize side effects.

Again, as with the oral forms, there is no solid evidence that the prophylactic administration of antiparkinsonian drugs prevents the

Table 1
Long-Acting Antipsychotics

Drug Class	Administration Route	Duration of Action (Weeks)	Average Dose
Phenothiazines			
Fluphenazine enanthate	IM	2	25-100 mg
Fluphenazine decanoate	IM	3	25-100 mg
Pipothiazine undecylenate	IM	2	100-150 mg
Pipothiazine palmitate	IM	4	50-300 mg
Thioxanthenes			
Flupenthixol decanoate	IM	2	12.5-50.0 mg
Diphenylbutylpiperidines			
Fluspirilene	IM	1	2-10 mg
Penfluridol	Oral	1	10-60 mg

occurrence of extrapyramidal side effects. Evidence is accumulating that for most patients who develop extrapyramidal side effects (and only 30% to 40% will) the administration of antiparkinsonian drugs for five days after an injection will control the side effects.[9]

No discomfort or irritation at the site of injection has been reported, although it is recommended that the site of injection be rotated.

There is no solid documentation to date to demonstrate that the prolonged administration of injectable psychotropic drugs produces any permanent alteration of liver, kidney, or bone marrow functions; nor does it produce ocular pigmentation or dermatologic discolorations.[10]

Finally, many patients will improve on the injectable drugs who did not improve on the oral form. A study by Curry and Lewis demonstrated this and also provided data as to the mechanism involved.[11] Curry and Lewis had taken 39 chronically hospitalized schizophrenics and treated them for one month with oral chlorpromazine. After a given dosage they collected blood samples and assayed chlorpromazine plasma levels. They continued the patients on the oral chlorpromazine for another week and then substituted an intramuscular dose for one of the oral doses. They collected blood samples and assayed chlorpromazine plasma levels again. Before disclosing the findings, they switched all the patients to an injectable neuroleptic and treated them for two more months and then evaluated the patients for clinical improvement. (The injectable used was fluphenazine decanoate, as there was no long-acting chlorpromazine; they had used chlorpromazine in the earlier phase because no method was available for determining fluphenazine levels.) Curry and Lewis found that of the 39 patients, 13 improved, 21 patients showed no change, and 5 patients deteriorated with injectable neuroleptic treatment. At this point, they examined their data on plasma levels of chlorpromazine following the oral administration and following the intramuscular dosage, grouping patients as to whether they had improved, deteriorated, or shown no change with the long-acting fluphenazine decanoate. They found that in patients who improved, the mean drug plasma level was 60% higher following the intramuscular dose than it was following the oral dose. In the patients who showed no change, the mean intramuscular drug plasma level was only 25% higher than the mean oral drug plasma level. And in those patients whose conditions deteriorated, the mean intramuscular drug plasma level was less than 20% higher than the mean oral drug plasma level. Curry and Lewis concluded that those patients who least effectively absorb oral chlorpromazine were those who improved most on the long-acting injectable fluphenazine, and vice versa. Curry and

Lewis speculated that individual differences exist in the capacity to absorb oral medication through the gastrointestinal tract and/or to metabolize it via the liver. They further speculated that a history of long use of psychotropic drugs may enhance a patient's ability to absorb and metabolize the orally ingested drugs. They cite this as rationale for trying an injectable form in a patient refractory to oral medication.

In considering the individual drugs, there is little to say about *fluphenazine enanthate* that does not apply to *fluphenazine decanoate*, the variant that seems to be replacing it. Therefore, only fluphenazine decanoate will be discussed, and fluphenazine enanthate differences will be cited.

Fluphenazine decanoate has a mean duration of activity of three weeks with an effective range of two to six weeks, and the enanthate has a mean duration of action of two weeks with a one- to four-week range of effectiveness. Both forms of the drug are used in the same dosage range: 25 to 75 mg in the acute stage, with dosages reduced to 12.5 mg for maintenance. Further dosage manipulation can be accomplished by altering the intervals between injections. Dystonic reactions may occur to each drug—usually within the first 48 hours (the enanthate is slightly more likely to cause them than is the decanoate). The 25-mg dose is most likely to cause extrapyramidal symptoms; with smaller and with much larger doses extrapyramidal symptoms occur less frequently and are of lesser severity. These symptoms occur with about the same frequency and intensity with the injectable forms as they do with oral forms and are easily treatable with any of the antiparkinsonian drugs. Antiparkinsonian medication on an as-needed basis suffices for many patients. Patients also may complain of a variety of side effects from both drugs, including akinesia, akathisia, insomnia, dizziness, blurred vision, tremors, and rigidity.

Two suggestions could guide application of these drugs. First, obtain a good drug history for the patient and his close relatives. A history of either good responsiveness or susceptibility to neurologic reactions in relatives augurs the same for the patient. Second, since fluphenazine decanoate is equally effective, longer-acting, less expensive, and produces fewer side effects than fluphenazine enanthate, there would seem to be few logical reasons to use the latter.

There is not too much in the literature about *flupenthixol decanoate*, but it has been tried in Europe (most extensively in Norway) and found to be similar to its phenothiazine analogues. It has a mean duration of action of two to four weeks, but it is somewhat more likely to produce extrapyramidal side effects than are fluphenazine enanthate and decanoate.

Oral pipothiazine is really just another phenothiazine, possessing clinical and adverse actions typical of this class of drug. There is nothing outstanding or unique about the drug. *Pipothiazine undecylenate* has a two-week duration of action following each injection. The average dose is 50 mg, and it has been used in doses of up to 250 mg. Clinically, the drug has shown itself as effective as fluphenazine enanthate, and it causes similar side effects. While the pipothiazine undecylenate can produce insomnia, it may often produce marked sedation. A number of investigators have reported severe depression (which required treatment with a tricyclic antidepressant) in schizophrenics who have taken the drug for several months, but this claim had also been made about the fluphenazine forms. The undecylenic form can cause hypotension, vertigo, and amenorrhea.

Pipothiazine palmitate is a longer-acting form and averages about four weeks' duration of action, with a two- to eight-week range of effectiveness. It, too, is administered in a sesame oil suspension of 25 mg/cc, but the average effective dose requires a 4 to 8 cc injection! The extrapyramidal reactions noted with the pipothiazine palmitate occur less frequently and are less severe than with the undecylenic. In addition to the side effects noted with the undecylenic, the palmitate may also cause restlessness, constipation, nausea, and vomiting. Changes in liver function tests have been noted (elevated SPGT and alkaline phosphatase), but no abnormal clinical signs associated with these changes were observed. There is one study that reports the drug useful in improving the behavior of autistic children.[5]

The two diphenylbutylpiperidines are the most interesting of the long-acting neuroleptic innovations. *Fluspirilene* is administered intramuscularly as an aqueous micronized suspension, and its duration of action is about one week. It requires no chemical conversion (ie, hydrolysis) to be active. It is used in dosages of from 1 to 10 mg weekly. While it does produce extrapyramidal symptoms, fluspirilene does not induce acute dystonic reactions as do all of the other drugs previously described. Furthermore, when extrapyramidal symptoms do occur (within 12 hours after an injection), they usually subside spontaneously within 48 hours. These symptoms can be further abated by use of an antiparkinsonian drug for two to three days after injection of the neuroleptic. Transient nausea, vomiting, mild hypotension, gastric discomfort, and fatigue have been noted shortly after injections.

Penfluridol, another diphenylbutylpiperidine, is the only one of the group of drugs discussed that is given orally, and it is effective for one week. It is a most useful drug for maintenance purposes (where excessive motor agitation is not a major target symptom), but it can also be used in acute states. The effective dose is 30 to 50 mg, and its effects are noted within a couple of hours. Other than showing extra-pyramidal symptoms, akathisia, trembling, and some drowsiness shortly after an injection, penfluridol is relatively free of side effects, and any side effects which do occur usually subside within two days. Penfluridol, like fluspirilene, rarely produces acute dystonic reactions.[12]

In addition to the long-acting psychotropics, a long-acting anti-parkinsonian drug, *dexetimide*, has also been developed which is effective for one week after administration.

These long-acting psychotropics are remarkably free of side effects when given for extended periods. Full blood counts, urinalyses, and renal function tests are essentially normal, even after years of continuous treatment with these drugs. The only significant hazard that is associated with continuous, prolonged use of these medications is tardive dyskinesia. There are indications, however, that the injectable psychotropic drugs produce less, or less persistent, tardive dyskinesia than do the orally administered neuroleptics. This is probably due to the fact that the injectable forms can be given in lower dosages.

We will see and hear more of these long-acting drugs. Used judiciously, they should significantly alter the manner in which pharmacotherapy is practiced. They should provide better treatment at a lower cost and with fewer adverse effects, and they may well supply us with tools for investigating the biochemical abnormalities that produce mental illness.

REFERENCES

1. Lewis, D.M., Curry, S.H., and Samuel, G.: Long-acting flu-phenazines in schizophrenia. *Br. Med. J.* 1:671-672, 1971.

2. Blackwell, B.: Drug deviation in psychiatric patients. In Ayd, F., Jr. (ed.): *The Future of Pharmacotherapy: New Drug Delivery Systems.* Baltimore: International Drug Therapy Newsletter, 1973, pp. 17-32.

3. Ayd, F.: Fluphenazine decanoate—another long-acting injectable phenothiazine neuroleptic. *Int. Drug Ther. Newsletter* 5:13-16, 1970.

4. Astrup, C. and Grimsgard, A.: A study of flupenthixol decanoate and pipothiazine undecylenate in schizophrenia. *Acta Psychiatr. Scand.* 50:481-491, 1974.

5. Brown-Thomsen, J. (ed.): Pipothiazine, pipothiazine undecylenate, and pipothiazine palmitate: clinical evaluation of new depot phenothiazines in the Nordic countries, experimental results and summary of world-wide clinical trials. *Acta Psychiatr. Scand.* 49 (suppl 241):1-138, 1973.

6. DiMascio, A.: The butyrophenones: an overview of their pharmacologic and metabolic properties. In DiMascio, A. and Shader, R.I. (eds.): *Butyrophenones in Psychiatry.* New York: Raven Press, 1972.

7. Freeman, H.: Controlled trial of penfluridol in acute psychosis. *Br. Med. J.* 1:442, 1972.

8. Bankier, R.G.: A comparison of fluspirilene and trifluoperazine in the treatment of acute schizophrenic psychosis. *J. Clin. Pharmacol.* 13:44, 1973.

9. Chien, C-P, DiMascio, A., and Cole, J.: Antiparkinsonian agents and depot phenothiazine. *Am. J. Psychiatry* 131 (1):86-90, 1974.

10. Villeneuve, A.: Some comments on long-acting neuroleptics. In Ayd, F., Jr. (ed): *The Future of Pharmacotherapy: New Drug Delivery Systems.* Baltimore: International Drug Therapy Newsletter, 1973, pp. 61-68.

11. Curry, S.H., Lewis, D.M. et al: Fluphenazine decanoate in patients absorbing oral chlorpromazine ineffectively. In Ayd, F., Jr. (ed.): *The Future of Pharmacotherapy: New Drug Delivery Systems.* Baltimore: International Drug Therapy Newsletter, 1973, pp. 53-60.

12. Kline, N.: Antipsychotics: new, longer-acting, safer agents. *Curr. Prescrib.* 7:48, 1976.

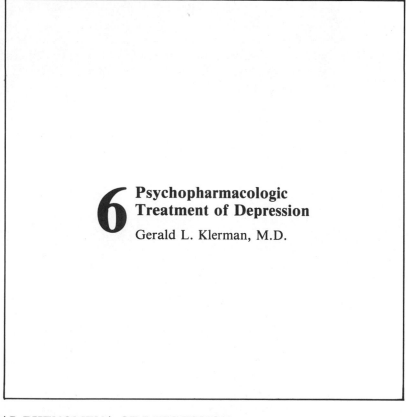

6 Psychopharmacologic Treatment of Depression
Gerald L. Klerman, M.D.

CLINICAL PHENOMENA OF DEPRESSION

It is important to understand the clinical phenomena of depression before one considers its treatment. Since the early part of this century, clinicians and investigators have grouped depression, mania, and related emotional states together as "affective disorders." In these disorders, the dominant feature is the disturbance of the patient's mood.[1] Descriptions of depression date back to ancient Egyptian, Greek, and Biblical texts, and excellent portraits of depressed individuals occur in Shakespeare's plays and in the romantic novels of the eighteenth and nineteenth centuries.

Depression, the most common affective disorder, is a syndrome in which persistent depression of mood is associated with feelings of worthlessness, guilt, helplessness, and hopelessness; anxiety, crying, suicidal tendencies, loss of interest in work and other activities; psychomotor retardation or agitation; impaired capacity to perform everyday social functions; and hypochondriasis. Bodily changes

63

include anorexia, weight change, and constipation. Mania is a less common, but dramatic, affective disorder. Some authorities also include anxiety and tension states among affective disorders, but current evidence suggests that these should be regarded separately.[2]

The term *depression* means different things to different clinicians and scientists, which leads to semantic confusion. For the neurophysiologist, depression refers to decrease in any electrophysiologic activity—for example, "cortical depression." To the pharmacologist, the word refers to drug actions which decrease the activity of the target organ; thus the central nervous system depressants include drugs like barbiturates and anesthetics. The psychologist uses the term depression for any reduction in optimal performance, such as slowing of psychomotor activity or reduction of intellectual functioning. For the clinical psychiatrist, professionals, and others in the mental health field, depression includes a wide range of changes in affective states—from the normal mood fluctuations of everyday life to severe melancholic, psychotic episodes.

Unfortunately, the use of the same term in a number of fields has perpetuated the view, and also the hope, that there is a single mechanism unifying the neurophysiologic, pharmacologic, and clinical phenomena. In the past, clinical psychiatric states were placed on a continuum based on degree of psychomotor activity. Manic excitement, presumably the result of excessive central nervous system excitation, represented one extreme and contrasted with depressive symptoms at the other, which were presumably caused by inhibition of generalized or specific central nervous system functioning. Moreover, the choice of treatment was determined by this approach and implemented the older classification of drugs affecting the central nervous system into stimulant and depressant categories, the drugs chosen being those which opposed the presumed central nervous system disorder. This "stimulant-depressant continuum" had been the classical approach for neuropharmacology. It was reasonable when the amphetamines and barbiturates were the principal forms of treatment.

The catecholamine hypothesis of affective disorder parallels the older view of a stimulant-depressant continuum. This theory has had great heuristic value, but it has not produced biochemical measures for diagnosis or assessment of clinical progress. Moreover, the complexity of actions of newer psychotropic drugs, particularly the phenothiazines and tricyclic antidepressants, contradicts the stimulant-depressant continuum model. The effects of lithium in preventing recurrence of both manic and depressive episodes suggest neurochemical processes common to elation and depression and the predisposition thereto. In the absence of firmly established neuro-physiologic, biochemical, or even psychodynamic mechanisms of causation or pathophysiology of affective disorders, assessment, diagnosis, and therapeutic decisions must necessarily be largely based on clinical criteria.

The Frequency of Depression

For the practicing clinician in mental health, the treatment of depression is a gratifying experience. Depressions are common, there are many treatments, and their results, for the most part, are good.

Depressions are the most common psychiatric condition that clinicians are likely to encounter in adult patients. Statistics indicate that the onset of a schizophrenic psychotic episode is most likely before the age of thirty. Epidemiologic studies in Great Britain, Scandinavia, and the United States show that perhaps 10% to 20% of all adults experience depressive episodes at some time.[3] However, only a minority of individuals with depressive symptoms and behavior patterns seek medical advice; and a much smaller proportion consult psychiatrists. Many distressed individuals do not seek medical care because of stigma, shame, or for other reasons; or they are "treated" by time alone or the psychotherapy of everyday life. Many more distressed individuals, however, suffer needlessly, often for prolonged periods.

Increased Frequency of Depression Among Women

Depressions occur more frequently among women than men.[4] The rates are about twice as high for women as for men: 25% for women and 10% for men. This differential, the subject of a lively controversy in epidemiology and research, is of great clinical interest as well.

The conventional explanation given for this difference is the hormonal changes which women experience at the premenstrual period, postpartum, and at the time of menopause. Hormonal factors have been the explanation discussed in most medical textbooks and in many of the women's journals. Another explanation holds that the difference is due not to hormonal factors, but to other confounding factors. Two such factors mentioned are the greater tendency of women to utilize all types of health services, and the use of alcohol by men. When a woman becomes depressed it is socially acceptable for her to complain and seek help from a health professional. Women present themselves to outpatient clinics more often, they are hospitalized more often, and they go to private practitioners more often than do men. Going to the clinic is not part of the stereotype of masculinity. It is more acceptable for a man to self-prescribe an agent such as alcohol—instead of frequenting the clinic, the man will frequent the bar or the cocktail lounge. This pattern has clinical importance, since a significant proportion of the man's (and the woman's occasional) use of alcohol to excess is part of a self-prescribed regimen for the relief of depression, anxiety, or a combination of the two. These trends may indicate that the health system works for women and that men are better off at the cocktail lounge; but since men die at a younger age than women, the male pattern might be better interpreted as maladaptive. Men who have depressive conditions are prone to come for treatment later in the course of the illness than women, after their symptomatology has become severe. Women are likely to request treatment earlier in the clinical episode, when their symptoms are less intense and more readily treated.

Many feminists believe the symptoms of depression reflect their low social status. They assert that feelings of fatigue, worthlessness, low self-esteem, and lack of interest are not just psychopathologic, but that they reflect the woman's reaction to second-class citizenship in our social order.

Distinguishing Normal Mood from Depressive States

Feelings of sadness, disappointment, and frustration are part of the human condition. The distinction between normal feelings and morbid depression is not always clear, and other affective phenomena may or may not be regarded as pathologic. The "acute depressive episode" refers to a clinically manifest symptomatic state as distinct from the depressive mood or affect.

All human beings experience fluctuations in their mood as part of the human evolutionary capacity inherited by all mammalian species, and particularly by primates. We have the biologic capacity to react to loss and to similar frustrations with changes in mood, phase, and posture. This is normal sadness.

One clinical difficulty arises in making the distinction between this normal mood (sadness or discouragement) and the clinical state of depression which merits therapeutic intervention. One cannot point today to any hard criteria to make this distinction. The distinction between the normal state and the clinical state is usually made on the basis of some combination of four criteria. First is intensity; we somehow feel that beyond a certain intensity a state is no longer normal. In clinical practice, different clinicians set the cut-off point at different intensities. Second is duration; if a mood continues for an excessively long time, it is of longer than normal duration. Third is the presence of an apparent precipitating event, such as a loss or disappointment. Fourth is the quality of the depression; features such as hallucinations, delusions, suicidal thoughts, severe weight loss, or onset of depression independent of an apparent precipitating event usually are considered signs of illness.

The Depression Syndromes

In addition to the dominant disturbances of mood, depressive illness usually involves some of the following features:

1) Impairment of bodily functioning: disturbances in sleep, appetite, sexual interest, autonomic nervous system functions, and gastrointestinal activity;
2) Reduced desire and ability to perform expected social roles in the family, at work, in marriage, in school, etc;
3) Suicidal thoughts or acts;
4) Disturbances in perception, cognition and reality testing, as manifested by delusions, hallucinations, confusion, etc.

Suicidal thoughts and acts and impairment of reality testing are relatively infrequent. Their presence usually indicates that the patient requires psychiatric attention.

These depressed states are identified by symptomatic and behavioral data; diagnosis on etiologic criteria, though much to be desired, is far from being realized in psychiatry in general, and in the affective disorders in particular. Etiologic processes are multiple and include genetic, biochemical, personality, stress and life events, and social background. Some depressions are caused by drugs, such as amphetamines or rauwolfia. In most affective illnesses, the etiology is an uncertain and varying combination of stress, personality, central nervous system changes in catecholamines, and other factors invoked to explain them. Current knowledge about etiologic processes is incomplete and indirect, therefore the symptomatic and behavioral features of the disorders relevant to diagnosis and treatment will be emphasized.

The depressed patient seldom experiences only one of the symptoms described. Most manifest depressed mood in close association with a number of other symptoms, the whole constellation being recognizable as a clinical syndrome.

Although there is no general agreement on the bases upon which the various depressive syndromes should be distinguished from one another, most clinicians and researchers recognize a variety of disorders. A number of dualistic distinctions have been proposed, including the "psychotic-neurotic," the "retarded-agitated," and the "primary-secondary," each of which has proved partially useful in clinical work.

Textbooks traditionally describe classifications of different types of depression: manic depression, unipolar, bipolar, endogenous, reactive, psychotic, neurotic, agitated, retarded. Most textbooks carry these stereotypic distinctions from one edition to the next. Actually, very few of the patients whom one sees in clinical practice correspond to one of these ideal types; one almost always sees a mixture of predisposition and precipitating event.[5]

It is important to do an accurate assessment of the symptoms and mood that the patient is experiencing and to get a thorough history of previous episodes. Of a large series of depressed patients, only about 15% will have truly psychotic depressions by the criterion that the episode is of such severity as to interfere with perception of reality, cognition, ego functioning, and reality testing. Less than 10% will have had a manic episode, but when the manic episode occurs, it forecasts a relatively serious long-term prognosis, because all patients with manic episodes are likely to have recurrences.

AVAILABLE TREATMENTS

We are quite fortunate in that there are many treatments available, the most impressive being time itself.

The Natural History of Depressions

In the natural history of the acute depressive episode, most patients get better. Time is on the clinician's side. In a follow-up study of 200 depressives carried out in New Haven in 1967, 80% of the patients were symptom-free at 10 months.[6] Most acute depressive episodes are self-limiting. There is debate as to whether this self-limitation is due to some internal biologic clock, or whether it is because having become depressed sets into motion the psychotherapy of everyday life.

When someone communicates to the family that they are depressed, the family, neighbors, professionals and nonprofessionals mobilize to come to the assistance of the patient. Often these changes are further steps toward the resolution of interpersonal disputes and other family conflicts which may have been the context in which the acute depressive episode occurred. Most depressive episodes never reach the professional but are treated by the support and counsel of the family, friends, general medical practitioners, the clergy, or social agencies.

The majority of depressed patients have a single depressive episode without recurrence. However, about 40% do experience recurrent episodes. If the history is of mixed manic and depressive episodes, the probability of recurrence approaches 90%. Consequently, the diagnosis of a manic episode also indicates high risk for the patient to experience recurrences. This consideration becomes important in the planning of long-term management of patients.[7]

Psychotherapy

In the usual general medical and psychiatric practice, drug therapy will be the procedure of choice. Reassurance and supportive psychotherapy are necessary for all patients, although intensive psychoanalytic treatment is seldom called for. Family and marital therapy may be helpful.

During hospitalization, group and milieu therapy are the settings where the here-and-now situation should be discussed. Occupation therapy and social therapy are both necessary in hospital treatment. These important therapeutic procedures can be mentioned here only briefly, although they are of the greatest value for the success of treatment, as is well-planned and systematic aftercare, which may continue for months or years.

Amphetamines and Psychomotor Stimulants

From a historic point of view, the amphetamines were the first drug treatment with any degree of efficacy and specificity for depression. The amphetamines were introduced into clinical practice in 1936 for the treatment of narcolepsy. It was soon observed that they had two other effects, and these led to their widespread clinical use. First, they produced a decrease in appetite; and second, they produced a transient, but real, elevation in mood. It was this capacity to elevate mood over short periods which led to their widespread use as a treatment for depression. In actual clinical practice today, the amphetamines have a very limited place, if any, in the treatment of most depressions. This limitation is due to three factors:

1) The clinical effect on mood is short-lived, seldom lasting more than 7 to 10 days.

2) Tolerance develops; the patient requires more and more of the drug to reach the desired endpoint, and this leads to the risk of habituation and dependence on the drug.
3) The drugs have significant side effects in relation to their benefits: jitteriness, irritability, and cardiovascular stimulation.

Because of the drawbacks listed above, amphetamines were combined with barbiturates and a search was launched for alternative stimulants. The nonamphetamine stimulant that has gained the widest use is methylphenidate (Ritalin). Methylphenidate also has a mood-elevating effect and is less likely to produce addiction. Its main use, however, is not in adult depressions but in the treatment of childhood learning disability with hyperkinesis.

There are other nonamphetamine stimulants—phenmetrazine (Preludin), pipradrol (Meratran), deanol—all having little value in the treatment of depression. Methylphenidate continues to have some place, perhaps as an adjunct. Interestingly enough, the combination of methylphenidate and a tricyclic seems to potentiate the antidepressant effect of the tricyclic by augmenting its metabolism.

Many patients experience an increase in anxiety, tension, and irritability with the amphetamines. Barbiturates have often been prescribed as adjunctive treatment, and several amphetamine-barbiturate combinations are marketed.

The principal objection to the use of amphetamines is the incidence of abuse and dependence. Tolerance develops rapidly and the dose is often increased by the patient. With prolonged use of amphetamines, toxic psychoses resembling paranoid states may occur. A true withdrawal syndrome, which includes fatigue, hyposomnalism, and increased rapid eye movement (REM) sleep, has been documented.

Electroconvulsive Therapy

The second major advance in the biologic treatment of depression came in 1940 with the introduction of electroconvulsive therapy. Convulsive therapy has been the subject of much controversy. There is little doubt that it has been, and in some instances continues to be, abused. Nevertheless, it still has an important place in an overall treatment program for depression. There is a small but significant proportion of patients (about 5% to 10%) who do not respond to other treatments, psychologic or pharmacologic, and for whom convulsive therapy has significant benefit. Convulsive therapy is of great value for patients with intense suicidal drive, in whom one does not wish to wait 5 to 15 days for drug treatment to take effect. Convulsive therapy is also of value for patients who have the unusual but dramatic syndrome of depressive stupor: they stop eating, stop talking, take to bed, and may become incontinent. The parallel symptomatologies of depressive and catatonic stupor often make clinical diagnosis difficult.

The major adverse effect of electroconvulsive therapy is memory loss, which, while rarely severe, is distressing to the patient. The effect usually lasts only a week or two and can be ameliorated by restricting the frequency of convulsions to 2 or 3 per week and by limiting to under 12 or 15 the total number of treatments in any course. An average of 7 to 10 treatments is usually sufficient. Electroconvulsive therapy tends to act more rapidly than drugs and may also be effective when drugs have failed.

While it is difficult to predict accurately which patients will respond, experience indicates that favorable results will be obtained with middle-aged and older patients or with those with a "psychotic" or "endogenous" depression. Electroconvulsive therapy remains a valuable and effective treatment for the severely depressed, for the actively suicidal, and for those patients whose medical condition contraindicates the use of drugs.[8]

Phenothiazines and Other Antipsychotics

The phenothiazines came into clinical use in the 1950s. They are still widely used in the treatment of depressions and have value in patients with intense agitation, insomnia, and delusions as part of their psychotic depression.[9] Thioridazine (Mellaril) is the only phenothiazine specifically approved by the Food and Drug Administration for the treatment of neurotic depression, although almost all the other phenothiazines—trifluoperazine (Stelazine), chlorpromazine (Thorazine), prochlorperazine (Compazine), fluphenazine (Prolixin)— are also prescribed. The phenothiazines can be readily combined with the tricyclics. The combination of perphenazine and amitriptyline is marketed in two forms, Triavil and Etrafon, both of which are widely used. Pharmacologic evidence indicates this combination to be effective. Interestingly enough, the addition of a tricyclic like amitriptyline reduces the amount of extrapyramidal side effects that patients might otherwise experience with perphenazine.

Reserpine is an antipsychotic, or neuroleptic, which is not of value in the treatment of depression. Reserpine is not much used anymore in psychiatry, but it still is of use in the treatment of hypertension. About 15% of hypertensives treated with reserpine will develop clinical depressions, and these depressions are often clinically indistinguishable from naturally occurring depressions.

MAO Inhibitors

Two significant advances in specific antidepressant drug treatment occurred almost simultaneously in 1957 and 1958 with the introduction of the monoamine oxidase (MAO) inhibitors and the tricyclic derivatives. The MAO inhibitors have had an inconsistent history in psychiatry: some of the original members of the group were developed in Germany as rocket fuels. They came into psychiatry when the two hydrazines iproniazid (which is an MAO inhibitor) and isoniazid (which is not an MAO inhibitor) were introduced into the treatment of tuberculosis. The paradox lay in that the patients who felt better were those on isoniazid. Some of the patients on iproniazid developed schizo-affective states and manic excitements, which led Crane and other psychiatrists who observed them to speculate that patients with depressions might benefit from the mood-stimulating effect of these drugs.[10] There has been a debate as to whether George Crane or Nathan Kline was the first to explore the psychopharmacologic effects of the MAO inhibitors. Regardless of who deserves the credit, these drugs are of value in the treatment of depression.

There are two factors which limit the clinical value of the MAO inhibitors, however, in comparison to that of the tricyclic compounds. First, they are less effective; and second, they are more toxic. Some MAO inhibitors produce liver toxicity; at least two of the MAO inhibitors, iproniazid (Marsilid) and pheniprazin (Catron), were withdrawn from clinical use due to evidence of secondary hepatitis. All MAO inhibitors can produce hypertensive episodes involving acute headaches, convulsions, coma, and even death.

In almost all controlled studies where MAO inhibitors such as tranylcypromine (Parnate) or phenelzine (Nardil) (the two MAO inhibitors currently available for prescription use in the United States) have been compared directly with the tricyclics like amitriptyline or imipramine, the tricyclics have come out ahead. That is, about 30% to 40% more patients improved with the tricyclics.[11] In conclusion, the MAO inhibitors are not as effective and are far more toxic than the tricyclics.

Nevertheless, in the past few years there has been a reevaluation of the status of the MAO inhibitors. A number of excellent studies have been conducted in the United States and in Great Britain which indicate the pendulum probably swung too far against the MAO inhibitors. Robinson and Nies from the University of Vermont report more effective treatment with the careful regulation of enzyme inhibition activity, made possible through newly devised means of measuring MAO inhibitor blood serum levels.[12] Patients who have either not responded to a tricyclic or who have anxiety and phobic symptoms in addition to depression seem to respond well to the MAO inhibitor phenelzine. There are similar reports from Great Britain that variously called "atypical," or "hysterical," depressions may show a good response to treatment with MAO inhibitor drugs such as phenelzine.[13]

In general, MAO inhibitors should not be the first drugs used with a depressed patient unless some combination of three conditions is met:

1) Generally, if the patient reports he did well with an MAO inhibitor in a previous depressive episode, it is highly likely he will do well with it again.

2) There seems to be an increased likelihood of response to MAO inhibitors if other members of the patient's family have also responded to that class of drug.

3) The patient must be intelligent and cooperative. This is extremely important, since in order to use the MAO inhibitors, the physician must be knowledgeable of their pharmacology and the patient must understand the principles involved and must cooperate with the prohibitions on certain foods and drugs. Moreover, the patient should be able to recognize symptoms of rising blood pressure—rapid pulse, headache, sweating, etc—and get to an emergency room immediately if these symptoms should occur.

Tricyclic Antidepressants

The next class of drugs introduced were the tricyclics, which have many proven advantages in the treatment of depressions. The tricyclics are efficacious in a wide range of depressions and they are relatively safe. These two features have led to widespread use by psychiatrists, internists, and general practitioners.[14] The tricyclic group includes six different compounds now marketed in the United States. The parent compound is imipramine (Tofranil). Amitriptyline (Elavil) is the most frequently prescribed compound. Nortriptyline (Aventyl), desipramine (Norpramin), doxepin (Sinequan), and protriptyline (Vivactil) are the other members of the class.

Research results indicate the following combination of symptoms predicts a good response to tricyclics, especially in patients over age 35: severe weight loss, psychomotor retardation or agitation, early morning awakening, suicidal thoughts, and feelings of pessimism. These symptoms are called "endogenous" or "psychotic" depressions in older textbooks. The more closely the patient fits the endogenous symptom picture, the better the predicted response to tricyclics.[15]

The range of clinical efficacy among the tricyclics is similar to that of the phenothiazines. The pharmacology and clinical actions of the various tricyclics are similar, but there are differences in dosage and side effects. Some of the tricyclics (eg, doxepin and amitriptyline) have sedative and hypnotic actions and therefore are of value to patients experiencing insomnia, agitation, or anxiety. When taken by a normal person, 100 mg of amitriptyline has about the same hypnotic effect as 100 mg of pentobarbital. These sedative-hypnotic properties are of value, as at least 60% to 70% of depressed patients exhibit insomnia and anxiety as part of their clinical syndrome.

At the other end of the spectrum are the stimulating tricyclics, of which protriptyline is the most potent; it is therefore not prescribed for patients who are anxious or agitated. This action may be useful, however, for depressed patients with retardation, apathy, or neurasthenia.

Patients on tricyclics will experience a wide range of autonomic effects early in treatment which may be discomforting, but which are seldom dangerous. These include dry mouth, blurred vision, and constipation. Occasionally, urinary retention and delayed ejaculation may occur. At high doses there may be difficulty with memory and concentration. The most serious side effects, however, concern the cardiovascular system.

Postural hypotension occurs with both the MAO inhibitors and the tricyclics. For patients who have cardiac disease, postural hypotension can be a problem, since it may precipitate cardiac or cerebrovascular accidents. The major potential cardiac danger with the tricyclics is the inducing of cardiac arrhythmias. This effect is probably related to the capacity of these drugs to influence catecholamine metabolism. Patients over the age of 40 or 45 who are being considered for treatment with tricyclics should have a thorough medical evaluation, including an electrocardiogram. If there is any evidence of cardiac irregularity, an internist should be consulted before these drugs are prescribed. The patient on tricyclic drugs should be instructed to seek medical attention immediately if irregular heartbeats or episodes of light-headedness occur.

The dosage range of the tricyclic compounds is wide. It is possible to start patients with a low dosage, 20 to 40 mg per day of imipramine or its equivalent, and gradually build up to 300 mg per day. A therapeutic response may require from one to two weeks of treatment and may not be maximal until the third or fourth week. If clinical response has not occurred within four to six weeks at an adequate and individualized dose, there is usually no point in continuing the drug and an alternative treatment should be considered.

Tricyclic drugs should not be discontinued suddenly. A period of gradual withdrawal is desirable, since symptoms of nausea, vomiting, malaise, and muscular pains occasionally occur as part of a mild withdrawal reaction. Current clinical practice is to withdraw the drug slowly three months or so after remission, while carefully observing the patient's reactions.

We still do not know the full range of depressed patients for whom tricyclics are useful. Initially they were recommended for so-called psychotic, retarded, and endogenous forms of depression. While these types do respond well, the tricyclics also benefit the neurotic forms, even those with milder symptoms and/or precipitating stress. The best recommendation is to select patients on the basis of symptoms of the syndrome discussed above, and to proceed with careful regulation of dose and observation for improvement or adverse effects.

Minor Tranquilizers

The minor tranquilizers—meprobamate and the diazepoxide derivatives—are widely used for depression because of their capacity to influence anxiety and insomnia. However, controlled studies of the chlordiazepoxide-diazepam series indicate that they have limitations for the treatment of depression.[16] Their effects are mainly short-term ones for anxiety or insomnia, and they do not lend themselves to use for more than four to six weeks because of habituation and the need to increase the dose. Also, an important distinction must be made regarding types of insomnia. Drugs such as chlordiazepoxide (Librium) and diazepam (Valium) are useful for patients who have trouble falling asleep, but they are less useful for patients who have early morning awakening—one of the cardinal signs of severe depression. Interestingly, patients with a high level of hostility and irritability, or those involved in tense interpersonal relations, do poorly on diazepam and chlordiazepoxide because of a tendency for disinhibition, leading to outbursts of anger or hostility, to occur.

ACUTE AND LONG-TERM TREATMENT

What does a clinician do when confronted by a patient with an acute or chronic depression? The first decision to be made concerns whether the patient needs medication. Many depressions do not require medication. Clinicians will follow different criteria with regard to the screening of patients and the selection of medications and dosages.

As a general rule, the fewer the social and interpersonal resources the patient has available, the more poorly he will do in all treatments, and the more prolonged will be his recovery from the depression.

If the clinician makes the decision to use medication, either immediately before or immediately after a trial of some other therapy, the tricyclics are the class of drug which has the greatest efficacy and the best relative margin of safety. If one chooses, one can use a minor tranquilizer like chlordiazepoxide, diazepam, or meprobamate, or a phenothiazine like thioridazine to treat anxiety and to facilitate a patient's sleep. An MAO inhibitor is not recommended as an initial drug, except under the circumstances outlined above.

If the patient does not show a clinical response to the first drug regimen within three to five weeks, he should be reevaluated with the following questions given careful consideration: (1) is he taking the medication, (2) is the dosage adequate? The median daily dose for outpatients will be between 100 and 150 mg of amitriptyline, or its equivalent; about 10% of patients will require more than 200 mg. At the other end of the spectrum, there are some patients who will respond to 50 or 75 mg.

If the patient does not respond to a tricyclic, the clinician can combine tricyclics with a phenothiazine or shift to an MAO inhibitor. If the patient is intensely suicidal or has other serious complications, hospitalization and/or electroconvulsive therapy should be considered. A logical treatment plan should be developed with an escalating sequence of intervention.

Long-term Treatment

Long-term treatment is currently the area of greatest interest in the therapeutics of depression. There has been a shift of concern from how to manage the acute episode to the long-term problems of the depressed individual.[17] Much of this interest has been stimulated by the advent of lithium, and some by the increased confidence of patients that they can get over the acute episode without hospitalization. There are three types of patients who require long-term treatment: (1) patients who relapse, (2) patients who have chronic depressions, and (3) patients who have recurrences.

Relapse It is widely believed that the acute depressed episode has an inherent time limitation. As mentioned earlier, follow-up studies show about 80% to 85% of patients asymptomatic at one year, with the average duration of the acute depressive episodes varying from 3 to 6 months. However, the path of recovery is not smooth and is subject to fluctuation. About half the patients will have a relapsing and fluctuating clinical course over the year. They may have occasional returns of insomnia, periods of irritability, difficulties in their inter-personal relations, and sexual problems that will wax and wane after the acute symptoms have subsided. Interestingly enough, a previous history of neurotic conflict predicts a relapsing course. Maintenance therapy is often useful with these patients, as is psychotherapy.

Chronic depressives　While 85% of patients were symptom-free at one year, 15% were not. This is a large group if one considers the total number of people suffering acute episodes. Robins and Guze reviewed 22 studies and found that an average of 15% of depressions have a chronic course.[18] Many of these chronically depressed patients are called "depressive characters." Their chronic depression becomes part of their life-style. The group includes the chronic hypochondriacal patient seen in medical clinics: the patient who wanders from ortho-pedics to endocrinology, to thyroid, to gastroenterology. Another is the bitter pessimist. With such patients, a careful history often reveals an acute depressive reaction a number of years earlier, such as an unresolved grief or disappointment. The acute episode was partially resolved, but did not completely remit, and the patient was left with the psychic scar of a chronic depression. Many such people persist for years in distress and desperation, making themselves and others miserable. Their symptoms may not be as severe as a suicide attempt, severe insomnia, or a 20-pound weight loss; rather, there will be bouts of irritability and subtle differences in work patterns and in sexual relations. Many depressed people present themselves with their sexual difficulties.

Depressed people are also poor parents. The depressed individual may appear inhibited in the expression of hostility outside the home, but his children report the anger and hostility they experience inside the home.

Recurring depression　A recurrence is distinguished from a relapse by the existence of an interval of well-being. As previously mentioned, most depressives get over their acute episode, but about 40% to 60% will have subsequent recurrences at some point in their lives. There are now six double-blind, placebo-controlled studies which demonstrate that lithium has value in the prevention of recurrences, and there are four studies on the value of maintenance tricyclics.[19] [20]

Maintenance treatment is not recommended for patients in their first recurrence. If there is a second recurrence, however, maintenance treatment should be considered. Patients with a history of mania or elation fall into the bipolar, or manic-depressive, group. For these patients, lithium is very effective in the prevention not only of the recurrence of a manic episode but of that of a depression as well. For the patient with multiple depressions, it is not clear whether to prescribe lithium or a tricyclic. About one third of patients on lithium will have some depressive symptoms. Lithium seems to be better at putting a ceiling on the highs; it makes a rather porous floor under the lows. Combinations of a tricyclic and lithium have been used and appear to be effective and safe.

CONCLUSION

We should emphasize the high incidence of depression in adulthood. There are a number of treatments of different degrees of efficacy available. For general clinical practice today, when the decision is made to use a drug, the tricyclics seem to be the best choice among available antidepressants. It is very important, however, to distinguish the treatment of the acute episode from the more difficult and challenging problem of planning for those patients who need long-term drug treatment for either frequent recurrences or for chronic depressive states.

In conclusion, depression is a common clinical condition, and its treatment is a very rewarding experience. For the most part, time is on the patient's and our side. The skillful use of available treatments can prevent suicide, facilitate a patient's return to a normal state, and make life much more gratifying for the patient and the family.

REFERENCES

1. Kraepelin, E.: *Manic-Depressive Insanity and Paranoia.* Edinburgh: Hogarth, 1921.

2. Prusoff, B. and Klerman, G.L.: Differentiating depressed from anxious neurotic outpatients: use of discriminant function analysis for separation of neurotic affective states. *Arch. Gen. Psychiatry* 30:302-309, 1974.

3. Klerman, G.L. and Barrett, J.E.: The affective disorders: clinical and epidemiological aspects. In Gershon, S. and Shopsin, B. (eds): *Lithium: Its Role in Psychiatric Treatment and Research.* New York: Plenum Press, 1973.

4. Weissman, M.M. and Klerman, G.L.: Psychotherapy with depressed women: an empirical study of content themes and reflection. *Br. J. Psychiatry* 12:55-61, 1973.

5. Klerman, G.L.: Clinical research in depression. In Zubin, J. and Freyhan, F. (eds.): *Disorders of Mood.* Baltimore: Johns Hopkins University Press, 1972.

6. Paykel, E.S. et al: Maintenance therapy of depression. *Pharmakopsychiatr. Neuro-Psychopharm.* 9:127-136, 1976.

7. Robins, E., Munoz, R., Martin, S. et al: Primary and secondary affective disorders. In Zubin, J. and Freyhan, F. (eds.): *Disorders of Mood.* Baltimore: Johns Hopkins University Press, 1972.

8. Klerman, G.L., Paykel, E.S. and Tonks, C.: Treatment of depression. In Conn, H. (ed.): *Current Therapy.* Philadelphia: W.B. Saunders Company, 1969.

9. Fink, M., Klein, D. and Kramer, J.: Clinical efficacy of chlorpromazine-procyclidine combinations, imipramine, and placebo in depressive disorders. *Psychopharmacologia* 5:27-36, 1964.

10. Crane, G.E.: Further studies on iproniazid phosphate, isonicotinilisopropylhydrazine phosphate, Marsilid. *J. Nerv. & Ment. Dis.* 124:322, 1956.

11. Davis, J.M., Schildkraut, J.J., and Klerman, G.L.: Drugs used in the treatment of depression. In Efron, D.H. et al (eds.): *Psychopharmacology: A Review of Progress, 1957-1967.* Washington, D.C: Government Printing Office, 1968, pp. 719-747.

12. Robinson, D.S., Nies, A. et al: The monoamine oxidase inhibitor phenelzine in the treatment of depressive-anxiety states: a controlled clinical trial. *Arch. Gen. Psychiatry* 29:407-413, 1973.

13. West, E.D. and Dally, P.J.: Effects of iproniazid in depressive syndromes. *Br. Med. J.* 1:1491-1494, 1959.

14. Klerman, G.L. and Cole, J.: Clinical pharmacology of imipramine and related antidepressant compounds. *Pharmacol. Rev.* 17:101-141, 1965.

15. Overall, J., Hollister, L., and Pennington, V.: Nosology of depression and differential response to drugs. *JAMA.* 195:946-48, 1966.

16. Covi, L., Lipman, R.S., Derogatis, L.R. et al: Drugs and group psychotherapy in neurotic depression. *Am. J. Psychiatry* 131:191-198, 1974.

17. Prien, R., Klett, C., and Caffey, E.: Lithium prophylaxis in recurrent affective illness. *Am. J. Psychiatry* 131:198-203, 1974.

18. Robins, E. and Guze, S.: Classification of affective disorders: the primary-secondary, the endogenous-reactive, and the neurotic-psychotic concepts. In Katz, M. and Shield, J. (eds.): *Recent Advances in the Psychobiology of the Depressive Illnesses.* Washington, D.C: U.S. Government Printing Office, 1972.

19. Davis, J.M.: Overview: maintenance therapy in psychiatry. II. Affective disorders. *Am. J. Psychiatry* 133:1-13, 1976.

20. Quitkin, F., Rifkin, A., and Klein, D.F.: Prophylaxis of affective disorders. *Arch. Gen. Psychiatry* 33:337-341, 1976.

7 Lithium Treatment of Atypical Manic-Depressive Illness

Bernard Levy, M.D.

INTRODUCTION

The beneficial effects of lithium in the treatment of acute mania and its use in the prophylaxis of recurrent manic or depressive episodes are now widely recognized. In addition, lithium can successfully treat a variety of atypical manic-depressive illnesses. Some investigators have reported sporadic successes with the use of this drug in the treatment of symptom complexes resembling schizophrenic illness, reactive depression, alcoholism, and sociopathic personality.[1] Yet these symptom complexes may actually be atypical manifestations of manic-depressive illness, and recognizing this is critical to developing the diagnostic acuity which will better differentiate classes of patients who will respond to treatment with lithium. One can establish a high level of awareness of the possibility of atypical manic-depressive illness by paying careful attention to family history and by keeping in mind that age-specific subgroups can regularly present with psychiatric manifestations not generally recognized as being part of the spectrum of manic-depressive illness. This perspective has been gained over the last 12 years in the course of supervising lithium treatment in over 1000 patients and of following their response to medication.* Many of these patients are often not recognized as belonging to the affective illness group but rather are thought to suffer from schizophrenic illnesses, reactive depressions, alcoholism, or sociopathic personalities.

Over 50 years ago, Adolf Meyer and two of his disciples, Leslie B. Hohman and Wendell Muncie, had recognized the many-faceted presentation of manic-depressive illness.[2] They noted that depression could start not only as a state of sadness but also as a paranoid state, depersonalization, perplexity, confusion, amorousness, or any other heightened and prolonged emotion. They strove to establish differential diagnosis of psychiatric illnesses primarily in order to be able to predict chances of recovery and to be able to distinguish affective illness from the more chronic and unremitting schizophrenic illnesses. Interest in Meyer's work was lost with the shift in American psychiatry to a psychodynamic orientation toward psychiatric illness. British psychiatry, however, has been more heavily influenced by Meyer's teaching and by the disease concept of psychiatric illness, and affective illness is a diagnosis made with much greater frequency there. The need for an understanding of the clinical issues that underlie these differences in practice has become compelling with the availability of specific therapy for the spectrum of manic-depressive illnesses. Currently in American psychiatry, patients with atypical manic-depressive illness are often mislabelled as schizophrenic, with the result that effective therapy is not considered.

ATYPICAL MANIFESTATIONS OF MANIC-DEPRESSIVE ILLNESS

The antimanic potential of lithium was first demonstrated by Cade, and then by Shou, in the early 1950s.[3][4] More than a decade later, Hartigan and Baastrup each demonstrated the usefulness of lithium in preventing depressive and manic episodes,[5-7] and in the last 10 years much effort has been devoted to demonstrating the effectiveness of lithium in classic manic-depressive illness. In 1968 it was recommended that lithium be tried in atypical cases if the illness were episodic and if there were a strong affective component.[8] Subsequently, Lipkin and his colleagues recognized that paranoid reactions could be manifestations of an affective illness, and they reported their experience with five cases successfully treated with lithium.[9] Other investigators have reported on lithium's effectiveness in other

---

*Bernard Levy: unpublished data.

conditions. It has been suggested that lithium is useful in epilepsy, recurring aggression, aggressive behavior in children and adolescents, sociopathic personality, mental deficiency, schizophrenia, periodic catatonia, premenstrual tension, and recurrent alcoholism. Much of this work is reviewed by Kline and Simpson.[1]

Yet most investigators do not consider the possibility that the symptoms they are studying in these disorders may be manifestations of manic-depressive illness. In order to identify those patients in whom a trial of lithium therapy may be beneficial, it is essential to recognize that manic-depressive illness may present in many forms besides those of retarded or agitated depression and elation. Frequently the symptoms of the illness obscure the underlying basic process, and several different types of symptomatology generally not recognized as affective illness may respond to lithium. The most common manifestations of atypical manic-depressive illness are acute psychosis in adolescence, recurrent paranoid psychosis, recurrent depressions in patients with extraordinary vocational success, alcoholism, and psychopathy.

Acute Psychosis in Adolescence

Acute psychosis in adolescence presents the greatest difficulty in diagnosis. Quite frequently the patient is thought to be suffering from a schizophrenic illness; but hallucinations and bizarre behavior are not sufficient evidence to establish a diagnosis of schizophrenia, as such symptoms are also seen in affective psychoses. It is also important to recognize that the ambivalence of adolescence compounds any psychosis occurring at that age, and that ambivalence is not necessarily pathognomonic of schizophrenia. Frequently the family history is very helpful in establishing a diagnosis. The physician should question the parents closely about evidence of affective illness in the family: episodes of depression, mania, suicide, or early retirement for emotional reasons. An acute onset, with a healthy premorbid state, also increases the likelihood that the adolescent has an affective disorder. Therefore, the psychiatrist should consider the possibility of manic-depressive illness in acute psychosis in adolescence, especially when the patient demonstrates strong emotions, even if these emotions are paranoid or bizarre. Additionally, if the psychosis clears completely, with no residual symptomatology, and then recurs months or years later, a diagnosis of manic-depressive illness is likely. Differential diagnosis is important, because lithium is the only available therapy specific to affective illness. Lithium has few side effects and adolescents frequently will tolerate it much more readily than they will the phenothiazines or other antipsychotic medications which tend to produce sedation and extrapyramidal symptoms. Furthermore, manic illness which first appears in adolescence has a greater tendency to recur than that which starts later in life, and lithium can prove extraordinarily helpful in preventing relapses. Generally, treatment should be maintained after remission has occurred, and the drug's continued use evaluated annually.

Recurrent Paranoid Psychosis

Paranoid psychosis may have an affective basis; often there is an underlying cyclothymic personality. Frequently the paranoia is more apparent than are the depressive symptoms. Paranoid ideation of acute onset and episodic nature frequently responds to lithium therapy.

Recurrent Depression in Patients with Extraordinary Vocational Success

We are accustomed to thinking of most mental illnesses as counterproductive to vocational success, but some patients with extraordinary vocational achievements are troubled on occasion by recurrent depressions. They work many hours a day with few hours of sleep, and many times this extra energy allows them to arrive at the top of their field. In many ways their life patterns may reflect a hypomanic state. However, they do have recurrent episodes of depression. These depressions have responded to antidepressant medication, and maintenance therapy with lithium has prevented their recurrence. The patients note that their old energy persists, and that they are less troubled by mood swings and depression. This freedom from mood swing and depression permits them to work more consistently and productively, and they are happier personally because the fear of possible recurrence is removed. While the possibility exists that lack of creativity and loss of energy might be related to lithium therapy, this author has not observed such an effect.

Alcoholism

While alcoholism is often a culturally derived or characterologic problem, there are people who use alcohol to treat the depression of recurrent affective illness. The sedation and insensibility of an alcoholic stupor relieves them momentarily of their depression. Only later, when the problems of alcoholism ensue, do they seek help. While they may at first appear to be similar to other alcoholics, careful inquiry reveals the depression which preceded the drinking. Lithium is not a specific treatment for alcoholism, but it has helped maintain sobriety in patients with this syndrome after they have undergone antidepressant drug therapy.

Psychopathy

The psychopathy of an acute manic episode which is manifested by giving away money or by sexual promiscuity is easily recognized; milder forms may be less easily diagnosed as manic-depressive illness. Erratic performance on the job, insufficient attention to details of work, extravagant promises, fantastic descriptions of past events and other distortions of the truth, and failure to meet responsibilities may all reflect a mood disturbance rather than a neurotic disorder. Again, the family history and a history of acute episodes are both helpful in establishing a diagnosis.

Rifkin et al have described a similar syndrome as an "emotionally unstable character disorder."[10] This syndrome is characterized by chronic maladaptive behavior patterns—such as truancy, poor work history, manipulativeness, and nonacceptance of reasonable authority—and depressive and hypomanic mood swings. They achieved success in ameliorating the symptoms with lithium in the majority of patients in a double-blind crossover study.[10] Unfortunately, they made no effort to separate out those who had clear-cut family histories and diagnoses of manic-depressive illness from those who might have been more accurately described as having character disorders. Perhaps their work will motivate others to attempt to replicate their findings and, in so doing, sharpen our diagnostic acumen.

On the other hand, it may be true that lithium is also useful for a spectrum of patients who are not manic-depressive but who simply have emotionally unstable characters. Currently the diagnosis "borderline personality" is much in vogue. Many of the patients so diagnosed fit the emotionally unstable character description and show an excellent clinical response to lithium.

TOXIC PSYCHOSES

While the tendency is to underdiagnose manic-depressive illness and to fail to recognize the multifaceted nature of this illness, there is one area where the tendency may be to overdiagnose. Due to an increase in illicit drug use and alcohol abuse, toxic psychoses are common. Many patients with these psychoses present in a state of hyperexcitability secondary to drug use, and their condition may be mislabelled as a manic episode. One way of avoiding this diagnostic error is to obtain a drug screen on all admissions and to be especially alert to any evidence of disorientation or other signs of an organic brain syndrome.

CONCLUSION

Lithium is among the most effective and least costly of psychiatric treatments for affective illness. The psychiatrist should be sensitive to the possibility of atypical syndromes, and a therapeutic trial of lithium may be indicated in doubtful cases. A favorable response to the medication may aid in establishing the diagnosis. Current evidence suggests that many more patients could benefit from lithium therapy than are currently being treated with it.

REFERENCES

1. Kline, N.S. and Simpson, G.M.: Lithium in the treatment of conditions other than the affective disorders. In Johnson, F.N. (ed.): *Lithium Research and Therapy.* New York: Academic Press, 1975, pp. 85-97.

2. Muncie, W.: *Psychobiology and Psychiatry.* St. Louis: C.V. Mosby Co., 1939, p. 291ff.

3. Cade, J.F.J.: Lithium salts in the treatment of psychotic excitement. *Med. J. Austr.* 2:349-352, 1949.

4. Schou, M. et al: The treatment of manic psychoses by the administration of lithium salts. *J. Neurol. Neurosurg. Psychiatry* 17:250-260, 1954.

5. Hartigan, G.P.: The use of lithium salts in affective disorders. *Br. J. Psychiatry* 109:810-814, 1963.

6. Baastrup, P.C.: The use of lithium in manic-depressive psychosis. *Comp. Psychiatry* 5:396-408, 1964.

7. Baastrup, P.C. and Schou, M.: Lithium as a prophylactic agent: its effect against recurrent depressions and manic-depressive psychosis. *Arch. Gen. Psychiatry* 16:162-172, 1969.

8. Levy, B.S.: A practicum for the use of lithium salts in affective psychoses. *JAMA.* 206:1045-1047, 1968.

9. Lipkin, K.M. et al: The many faces of mania. *Arch. Gen. Psychiatry* 22:262-267, 1970.

10. Rifkin, A. et al: Lithium carbonate in emotionally unstable character disorder. *Arch. Gen. Psychiatry* 27:519-523, 1972.

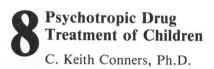

8 Psychotropic Drug Treatment of Children

C. Keith Conners, Ph.D.

Systematic studies of drugs in children have been made since the early 1930s—before studies of drugs in adults. Even before then, sedatives and hypnotics were used for calming difficult babies. On the whole, however, until 10 years ago therapy in children has reflected a predominantly psychodynamic approach. The approach to the use of drugs has been rather conservative, and recent debates have questioned the advisability of using drugs in children at all. The therapist, therefore, finds himself threading his way between pharmacologic conservatism and therapeutic nihilism. However, the literature does contain definite indications for the use of psychotropic drugs in treating children.

INFLUENCE OF ATTITUDES

There are some important limiting factors and general considerations which affect the clinical use of these therapeutic agents in children. The first variable influencing drug treatment is the attitude of the physician. Pediatricians, child psychiatrists, adult psychiatrists, and

86

general practitioners each use drugs quite differently. Surveys have shown that the type and dosage of drug used with children vary as a function of the training of the physician. Unfortunately, physicians tend to dichotomize along the lines of organic and psychodynamic approaches: on the whole, child psychiatrists tend not to use drugs; pediatricians, who are more "organically" oriented, tend to use them more frequently. We know that physicians who use drugs half-heartedly achieve poor results, either because their attitude affects the quality of response directly, or because they employ homeopathic doses. Compliance in the taking of drugs is a major problem with children, and here the attitude of the physician will have a direct impact on the extent to which the child receives the indicated dose, at least in an outpatient setting.

Of course, dosage of these drugs is different in children than in adults and may be a more critical determinant of effect. Therefore, in prescribing for children one has to be very familiar with the ranges of therapeutic efficacy. The most experienced practitioners and researchers in child psychopharmacology, though, typically report dosage values very much in excess (on a mg/kg basis) of those recommended in the package insert or in *Physician's Desk Reference (PDR)*, (except, possibly, in the case of the more potent piperazine phenothiazines).

Second, the attitude of the family is quite important; studies have shown that there are medication-accepting and medication-rejecting families.[1][2] It is incumbent upon the therapist to notice whether the parents have an anti- or pro-drug bias and to take this into account in deciding whether or not to use drugs. For example, if a family has had a prior experience with a child who has abused a drug, this may seriously limit their ability to follow the recommendations for psychotropic drug use. Similarly, parental doubts (which can be easily elicited) raised by sensationalistic newspaper articles can totally defeat an otherwise sound treatment plan.

A wish by the family to focus on some obscure organic etiology is not uncommon, and here it is necessary to be sensitive to the parents' covert abdication of responsibility for the child's illness, and to their antipsychologic attitudes. The best rule to remember is that all psychiatric complaints in children require psychologic methods of management in addition to other therapies. The drugs do not cure or educate; nor do they undo the basic causes of the disorder. In all cases, drugs are given for symptomatic treatment. Parents must be helped to see that they themselves are not the sole cause of the child's behavioral difficulties and that drugs are not the sole cure. Often some direct improvement with drug therapy will restore the parents' interest in discovering how they might better help their child. For example, frequently parents who are skeptical at first about the use of drugs are much encouraged when they discover that the drugs change their child's behavior, and that there is, in fact, something in the child, too, which is responsible for his problem. They now feel less guilt and are freer to better see their own role in the child's problems.

For children with the most severe pathology (such as organic retardation, hyperactivity, or psychosis) drugs frequently make the difference between staying at home and being institutionalized. Whether it is better for the child to stay home depends, of course, upon his family.

Third, one has to be aware of the attitude of the child. Most children will accept medication without a fuss if they're convinced that it will help them and if the adult role models are supportive and accepting. It is important, however, that those children who are able to understand be given some explanation, otherwise they may attribute a number of idiosyncratic rationales to the pills (eg, considering them "smart pills" or "stupid pills"). With most children, a matter-of-fact approach—"These medicines may help you to be more in charge of yourself," or, "They won't take away your school problems, but if you want to do better in school you may be able to"—is the most effective.

PHENOTHIAZINES

Shortly after the introduction of chlorpromazine for adults, use of the phenothiazines in children was reported on by Bender and by Freedman.[3][4] These early reports of noncontrolled studies gave uniformly positive pictures of the effects of phenothiazines in a variety of psychiatric disorders, including enuresis, reading disability, autism, schizophrenia, and sexual disorders.[1] Most of these claims have not been validated on subsequent examination, and the extensive use of the phenothiazines in controlling severely agitated institutionalized retardates has become one of the great scandals of modern therapeutics. It has become evident that children have been maintained for years on very high dosages of phenothiazines without regard to the drugs' effects on developmental status and cognitive function.[5][6]

No firm relationship has been established between any psychiatric diagnosis in children and the particular efficacy of the phenothiazines.[2] Rather, these drugs tend to be used for all diagnoses in children with intractable and severe symptomatology. In general, the more potent piperazine drugs are used with the more severely schizophrenic, autistic, or organically impaired children, particularly those who become sedated with chlorpromazine and require the presumedly stimulating effects of the piperazines to counteract apathy, withdrawal, and retarded speech. There is no firm evidence that the so-called stimulating phenothiazines do anything more than produce general restlessness or akathisia.[7] There is general agreement now that the phenothiazines should be used only after an adequate attempt at environmental or psychotherapeutic management has failed, or as a form of crisis intervention to facilitate educational or therapeutic efforts. Recent developments with behavior modification, for example, offer alternatives to the use of these drugs in many cases.

Dosage

One begins treatment, as with adults, with the lowest recommended dosage and increases this gradually over a period of weeks. There is greater variation in individual dosage requirements among children than among adults, and there are no firm rules as to dosages for different ages (whether this wider variation is due to differences in the maturation of the enzyme induction systems of the kidneys and liver is not known). Retarded schizophrenic children may tolerate larger doses of trifluoperazine or fluphenazine than will less impaired older children, and both Fish and Engelhardt have reported improvement in motor skills, social responsiveness, and language with such treatment.[8] [9] (This is about as close as one comes to a specific indication for the phenothiazines.) The adult dose, adjusted strictly for body weight, may be as much as two to five times too high for these children, so caution is advised in selecting the proper dosage. (See Table 1)

Adverse Effects

There is a high incidence of dystonic effects reported with the use of phenothiazines in children, and small doses of the piperazines may actually cause irritability, agitation, or dyskinesia.[10] Table 2 presents a description of some common side effects caused in autistic schizophrenic children in a number of trials. The most common side effect is lassitude and drowsiness, but it may frequently be a mistake to discontinue the drug early in treatment, as this side effect tends to disappear before long. Extrapyramidal symptoms range from mild tremors to severe parkinsonism, and the most disturbing side effect is the syndrome of dyskinesia, which includes torticollis, aphonia, and

Table 1
Phenothiazine Usage with Children

Generic Name	Recommended Oral Dosage			PDR	Status (PDR)*	Remarks
	Shaw & Lucas	Engelhardt et al	Chess			
Chlorpromazine	*5 to 12 years:* 75-300 mg/day; *over 12:* 75-1000 mg/day	81-496 mg/day; mean = 214 mg	5-100 mg/day	*Outpatients:* 0.5 mg/kg 3 or 4 times per day prn; *severe behavior disorders or psychotic conditions:* 50-100 mg daily; *older children:* 200 mg or more daily	1	
Promazine	*5 to 12 years:* 75-300 mg/day; *over 12:* 75-1000 mg/day			Not listed	0	
Triflupromazine hydrochloride	*5 to 12 years:* 30-100 mg/day; *over 12:* 50-150 mg/day			Not listed	0	
Thioridazine	*5 to 12 years:* 30-300 mg/day; *over 12:* 75-800 mg/day	50-791 mg/day; mean = 289 mg	1-15 mg/day	*2 to 12 years:* 0.5-3.0 mg/kg/day; *moderate disorders:* 10 mg 2 or 3 times per day; *severe disorders:* 25 mg 2 or 3 times per day	1	Not intended for children under 2 years of age
Trifluoperazine	*Under 12 years:* 1-20 mg/day; *over 12:* 4-40 mg/day	7-57 mg/day; mean = 35 mg	1-15 mg/day	1 mg once or twice a day	1	For children aged 6 to 12 who are hospitalized or under close supervision

Drug	Dosage (under/over 12)	mean		Rating	Notes
Perphenazine	*Under 12 years:* 2-16 mg/day; *over 12:* 6-64 mg/day		*Neurotic anxiety and tension states:* 2-4 mg 3 times per day; *moderately disturbed non-hospitalized patients:* 4-8 mg 3 times per day; *hospitalized psychiatric patients:* 8-16 mg 3 times per day	2	Not recommended for children under 20 lbs. in weight or less than 2 years of age
Prochlorperazine	*Under 12 years:* 5-30 mg/day; *over 12:* 15-75 mg/day	7-50 mg/day; mean = 20.3 mg	*2 to 12 years:* Starting dose is 2.5 mg 2 or 3 times per day (no more than 10 mg the first day); *ages 2 to 5:* total daily dose usually does not exceed 20 mg; *ages 6 to 12:* total daily dose usually does not exceed 25 mg	1	
Fluphenazine hydrochloride	*Under 12 years:* 1.0-7.5 mg/day; *over 12:* 2.5-20.0 mg/day	19-24 mg/day; mean = 12.5 mg	0.25 to 3.00 mg daily in divided doses	1	Oral dosages as high as 10 mg daily have been used in some older children

SOURCES: Shaw, C.R. and Lucas, A.R.: *The Psychiatric Disorders of Childhood.* 2d ed. New York: Appleton-Century-Crofts, 1970, p. 443.
Engelhardt, D.M., Polizos, P., and Margolis, R.A.: The drug treatment of childhood psychosis. In Smith, W.L. (ed.): *Drugs, Development and Cerebral Function.* Springfield, Ill: Charles C Thomas, 1972, pp. 224-234.
Chess, S.: *An Introduction to Child Psychiatry.* 2d ed. New York: Grune & Stratton, 1969, pp. 234-242.
Physician's Desk Reference. 31st ed. Oradell, N.J: Medical Economics Company, 1977.
*0 = no reference to children under 12; 1 = recommended for children under 12; 2 = not recommended for children under 12.

dysphagia. These side effects may be less apparent in disturbed children precisely because of their inability to verbalize. There is good reason to believe that the incidence of these side effects is very much underestimated.[2]

Recent reports indicate that the syndrome of tardive dyskinesia seen in adults may also appear in children upon withdrawal of phenothiazines.[11] In adults this syndrome is usually characterized by involuntary movements of the lips, mouth, tongue, and at times by bizarre movements of the trunk or extremities. While lateral jaw movements, tongue thrusts, and smacking of the lips are common in adults with tardive dyskinesia, these actions are much less prominent in children, who demonstrate more bodily movement symptoms. McAndrew reports on a retrospective survey of 125 inpatient children aged 4 to 16, and all of the children exhibited involuntary movements, as well as akathisia and general restlessness, upon drug withdrawal.[12] This is a rather frightening phenomenon because this syndrome in adults is often associated with some irreversible neurologic changes. In McAndrew's patients, however, changes tended to be reversible upon reintroduction of the drug. Nevertheless, this certainly suggests caution. In general, the low-dosage, high-potency phenothiazines tend

Table 2
Phenothiazine Side Effect Data for Five Single-Blind Studies

	Chlorpro-mazine	Thiorida-zine	Trifluo-perazine	Prochlor-perazine	Fluphena-zine
Number of trials	12	24	14	7	28
Number of trials with positive treatment emergent symptoms	7	17	9	3	19
Number of complaints					
Adverse behavioral effects	5(36)	16(12)	10(20)	3(23)	19(19)
Lethargy	2(14)	4(3)	2(4)	1(8)	8(8)
Increased appetite	0	46(35)	8(16)	1(8)	14(14)
Weight gain	1(7)	7(5)	3(6)	1(8)	10(10)
Gastrointestinal symptoms	0	0	0	3(23)	0
Anorexia	0	1(1)	0	2(15)	4(4)
Extrapyramidal symptoms	6(43)	7(5)	28(55)*	1(8)	33(34)
Genitourinary symptoms	0	47(36)	0	1(8)	10(10)
Photosensitivity	0	4(3)	0	0	0
Total complaints	14	132	51	13	98

SOURCE: Engelhardt, D.M., Polizos, P., and Margolis, R.A. The drug treatment of childhood psychosis. In Smith, W.L. (ed.): *Drugs, Development, and Cerebral Function.* Springfield, Ill: Charles C Thomas, 1972, p. 230.
NOTE: Numbers in parentheses represent percentages of total complaints.
*This figure is an underestimate, since 6 of the 14 children received procyclidine hydrochloride prophylactically and exhibited no extrapyramidal symptoms.

to be the worst offenders. That there are occasional reports of blood dyscrasias with phenothiazines suggests that weekly blood counts are probably a good idea—at least in the early part of therapy, since the effect, if it occurs, tends to develop early.[7]

Trials of phenothiazines in both animals and children have provided unequivocal evidence that these drugs are quite capable of impairing cognitive function.[6] Even rather low doses of phenothiazines will have an adverse effect on concept-formation tasks. Obviously there is a cost-benefit problem here. If control of severe agitation can only be gained at the cost of some impairment of sensation, concentration, and thinking, then one might have to pay that price. One should be aware, however, that there is such a price so that these drugs are not used lightly in the treatment of minor behavior problems.

OTHER MAJOR TRANQUILIZERS

Among the most effective of the other major tranquilizers is haloperidol, a butyrophenone. Haloperidol has been used quite widely in Europe for the treatment of agitation in schizophrenic, autistic, and organic disorders in children and adolescents, and it is often used effectively with adolescents who do not respond well to phenothiazines. It acts more quickly than the piperazines (such as fluphenazine) in the control of motor behavior and social disruptiveness.[12]

There is one rather obscure syndrome for which haloperidol is apparently a specific treatment: Gilles de la Tourette syndrome, whose etiology is not well understood. This is a bizarre syndrome involving an oral tick; the child usually barks like a dog and mouths obscenities in a nonstop fashion.

Side effects and toxicity with haloperidol are about the same as with the other major tranquilizers. The only important caveat with haloperidol is that one should be cautious when using this drug in conjunction with imipramine or in patients with seizure disorders, because it may potentiate the toxic effects of imipramine (sometimes to dangerous levels), and it appears to lower the seizure threshold (as do the phenothiazines).

The thioxanthene derivatives, such as thiothixene, have not been sufficiently studied, although one report suggests that cyclothymic retardates do well with this drug.[13] Another thioxanthene, chlorprothixene, is about as effective in controlled trials as is thioridazine, but it is less sedating in effect. However, these have not been used very much, and very few people in this country have experience with them.

MINOR TRANQUILIZERS

The minor tranquilizers are also known as antianxiety drugs (see Table 3). These have been used very extensively in outpatient treatment of children with a variety of symptoms, including school phobias, night terrors, anxiety attacks, enuresis, encopresis, insomnia, muscular tension, ticks, and hypochondriasis, and also in depressed and sexually precocious children. Despite this very wide range of use, however, there is a marked discrepancy between their success in controlled trials and their success in uncontrolled trials, and this raises some suspicions. Lack of careful diagnosis and of standardized methods of assessment is very common, and one should be skeptical about the efficacy of minor tranquilizers such as chlordiazepoxide and diazepam with most children.

Barbara Fish has conducted many trials of diphenhydramine (Benadryl) in children under seven who are anxious, irritable, or impulsive, or who in fact show the hyperkinetic behavior syndrome.[14] She recommends that because it is so well tolerated, diphenhydramine be the drug of first choice in younger hyperactive children. The extensive use of diphenhydramine by pediatricians is probably justified, although there have not been any controlled trials.[15]

Table 3
Minor Tranquilizer Usage with Children

Generic Name	Dosage	Status*	Remarks
Chlordiaz- epoxide	5 mg 2 to 4 times per day (may be increased in some children to 10 mg 2 or 3 times per day)	1	Not recommended for children under age 6
Diazepam	1.0-2.5 mg 3 or 4 times per day initially; increase gradually as needed and tolerated	1	
Meprobamate	100-200 mg 2 or 3 times per day	1	Not recommended for children under age 6
Tybamate	20-35 mg/kg/day in 3 or 4 equally divided doses	1	Not recommended for children under age 6
Hydroxyzine	*Under 6 years:* 50 mg daily in divided doses; *over 6 years:* 50-100 mg daily in divided doses	1	Pharmacologically classified as antihistamine
Diphenhy- dramine	5 mg/kg/day in 3 or 4 divided doses; daily dose not to exceed 300 mg	1	Pharmacologically classified as antihistamine

SOURCE: *Physician's Desk Reference.* 31st ed. Oradell, N.J.: Medical Economics Company, 1977.
*0 = no reference to children under 12; 1 = recommended for children under 12; 2 = not recommended for children under 12.

The use of the minor tranquilizers for mild spasticity and muscular tension is also probably justified on the basis of available evidence.

It has been reported that, as with adults, the use of drugs such as chlordiazepoxide in children may actually disinhibit aggressive and assaultive behavior;[16] so again, one should be cautious about using these drugs with acting-out, aggressive adolescents.

TRICYCLICS

Several controlled and partially controlled reports have appeared on the use of the tricyclics in children.[17] Though not currently recommended for use with children under 12, they appear to have some value in the symptomatic control of persistent enuresis (that is, in children who do not show an organic cause of the enuresis, and where enuresis has been present from the beginning).[2] Tricyclic drugs have also been employed in the treatment of encopresis, depression, and hyperkinetic impulse disorders.[2] While clearly not the drugs of initial choice, imipramine and amitriptyline appear to provide a useful alternative when other treatments have failed. The use of these drugs in depressive states in adolescence has not been well studied in the United States, but European studies indicate that they are beneficial.[18] Extensive trials with hyperkinetic children suggest that the antidepressants are as good or better than the stimulants in controlling this disorder.[19-21]

CHILDHOOD DEPRESSION

A rather neglected area in child psychopharmacology is the recognition and treatment of depressive states. Except for the very early kind of anaclitic splits (or the hospitalism syndrome) in young children, most American child psychiatrists do not believe there is such a thing as endogenous depression in children. European psychiatrists, however, who have looked at this matter rather thoroughly (especially since the introduction of lithium), believe that endogenous depressions do occur in children, though clinical manifestations may differ. Though alternating mania and depression do not appear to occur before the age of 10, reports as early as Kraepelin's suggest that such cyclothymic behavior does occur in younger children.[22] One first sees a rather sudden change in personality, usually of a depressive nature. One also finds a high incidence of affective illness in the parents, especially the mother. It has been shown that the siblings and children of bipolar depressive patients also have a very high incidence of affective illness.[23] There is thus a reasonable genetic basis for believing that endogenous bipolar depression, without the mania, occurs in children.

The depression is easily confused with a variety of other disturbances (eg, schizophrenia) because of the presence of psychotic elements, stupor, organic brain syndromes, or hyperkinesis. When these conditions fail to respond to other treatments, including psychotherapy and stimulant drugs, lithium carbonate may have a rather miraculous effect.[23-25] Although not, of course, a drug to be used indiscriminately, lithium may be worth a trial in some severe disorders when one suspects an endogenous type of depressive analog of adult affective disease.

TREATMENT OF HYPERKINESIS
Psychomotor Stimulants

The stimulants have the longest history of use in child psychiatry. Their action is often immediate and rather dramatic, though it may be short-lived. While they may provide fairly dramatic effects on behavior, perception, and intellectual function, the diagnosis must be exact because, of course, hyperactivity is a symptom in many other disturbances besides the hyperkinetic behavior syndrome.

Recent studies indicate that children who do not exhibit psychopathology but who have attentional defects with or without hyperactivity also show significant benefit with these agents.[26] For example, children with a reading disorder based upon a defect in the attentional system may show rather striking improvements with treatment with stimulants. Of course, there are many other kinds of reading disorders, and this is not a general prescription. Greater benefits do seem to be obtained by those children with a higher incidence of hyperkinetic signs.

Recent work by Millichap indicates that stimulant drug effects are much more marked in those children who show choreiform movements and left-right confusion.[22] There is also evidence from Satterfield's laboratory that children who have an excess of power in the lower frequency bands of the electroencephalographic spectrum are more likely to respond well to stimulants such as methylphenidate, dextroamphetamine, and levamfetamine.[28] A relatively new addition to our armamentarium for treating children with minimal brain dysfunction is magnesium pemoline, which appears to be a reasonably effective stimulant drug.[29] [30] It is not quite as potent as amphetamine or methylphenidate, but it seems to produce effects which last somewhat longer than the other stimulants, and it can therefore be given in single daily doses—a distinct advantage in treating outpatient children who have great difficulties in compliance.

There is some evidence that levamfetamine may be more effective than dextroamphetamine in more aggressive hyperkinetic children[26] and that this clinical variance derives from the subtle difference in optic isomers of the drugs. The variance in response to different optic isomers of amphetamine suggests a difference in the ability of their compounds to affect catecholamine receptors in the brain, and this suggests that aggressive hyperkinetic children may differ from happy-go-lucky hyperkinetic patients in some basic biochemical mechanism.[26]

The most common side effects of the stimulants are insomnia and anorexia, and again, these tend to diminish over a two-week period. With adjustment of dosage over a four- to six-week period, less than 5% of the children should experience persistent anorexia or insomnia. One of the side effects that is most perplexing and often most trouble-some to the physician (because parents get worried) is the so-called amphetamine look: the face may be pale and drawn, with bags under the eyes. The parents will swear that the child is about to die of some ominous disease, and they will want to take him off the drug, when in fact this is a local, peripheral effect and of no demonstrated significance.[31]

Few long-term studies have been reported with these drugs. Although they have been considered very safe over the years, reports of a growth-inhibiting effect by Safer et al give some cause for concern.[23] In looking at that data, one should remember that, although statistically significant, the changes reported were quite miniscule. One must consider too that two other laboratories have failed to confirm Safer's findings,[26] and that the doses at which this has been noted to occur are relatively high: it was the high-dose methylphenidate and amphetamine subjects that showed some apparent growth retardation. Further, there is reason to suspect that the control subjects in Safer's studies were in fact different in weight and/or height from the experimental subjects to begin with. Also, subjects in the amphetamine treatment study were those children whose parents accepted the treatment; therefore, they were likely to be the ones with severe symptoms. It is also possible these more severely impaired children were more likely to have had low birth weight and to have shown a different growth curve. Although this kind of retro-spective study leaves some important questions, one ought to consider the possibility of growth retardation before using these drugs in high doses over a long period.

Table 4 presents the recommended dosages for the stimulants according to *PDR*, but experience largely shows that the effective ranges are somewhat higher than those given here. Some children

98

function quite well with the single morning dose, while others require an afternoon dose in order to avoid deterioration in behavior at school. There is considerable disagreement as to whether one ought to give these children drug holidays on the weekends or during school vacation. This seems to be a decision one makes on the basis of the total adjustment pattern of the child. If he falls apart on the weekend, fights with his siblings and all the neighbors, and tears the house apart, a drug holiday is obviously contraindicated. On the other hand, if his symptoms are mainly school related, and if he acts poorly only under the stress and confinement of the classroom, then one would consider a weekend drug holiday appropriate.

There are a number of ethical issues associated with the use of the stimulants which deserve discussion. There is no question that injudicious use of the stimulant drugs has become something of a major problem. However, it's also clear that the kind of sensationalism in the newspapers and the indictment of this form of treatment as a form of behavior control is exaggeration, if not absolute

Table 4
Stimulant Drug Usage with Children

Generic Name	Dosage	Remarks
Amphetamine sulphate	*Range:* From 5 to 40 mg per day. Some older children may require more than 40 mg for optimal response; *3-5 years:* start with 2.5 mg daily; dosage may be raised by increments of 2.5 mg at weekly intervals until optimal response is obtained; *6 years and older:* start with 10 mg once or twice daily; dosage may be raised by increments of 10 mg at weekly intervals until optimal response is obtained	Not recommended for use in children under 3 years of age
Dextroamphetamine sulphate	*3-5 years:* Start with 2.5 mg daily; dosage may be raised by increments of 2.5 mg at weekly intervals; *6 years and older:* start with 5 mg once or twice daily; dosage may be raised by increments of 5 mg at weekly intervals	Not recommended for use in children under 3 years of age
Methylphenidate hydrochloride	*6 years and older:* Start with 5 mg before breakfast and lunch with gradual increments of 5-10 mg weekly. Daily dosage above 60 mg is not recommended. If improvement is not observed after appropriate dosage adjustment over a one-month period, the drug should be discontinued.	Not recommended for use in children under 6 years of age

SOURCE: *Physician's Desk Reference.* 31st ed. Oradell, N.J.: Medical Economics Company, 1977.

absurdity. Satterfield tells a story in refutation of the contention that these children become little automatons because they are given a "behavior-controlling" drug. He tells of a 10-year-old boy with severe hyperkinesis who became essentially normal with drug treatment and who proceeded to get up a successful class petition to have the school-teacher fired.* Here he presents a good example of a child being made capable of making his own decisions. The drug does not *make* him do anything at all; it simply gives him the freedom to choose, which he did not have before.

Other Therapies

As far as other somatic therapies are concerned, insulin therapy has never been proven to be of any value, electroconvulsive therapy in children is seldom used these days, and the recent fad use of mega-vitamins has not been shown to have any definite value. Although the latter may have a profound placebo effect, there is no evidence that megavitamins in fact do anything specific.

The role of food, food additives, and food dyes in the promotion of behavior disorders in children is currently being investigated. Feingold noted improvement in some adult patients' psychiatric symptoms when he treated their allergies to salicylates.[33] This improvement was noted when he took them off not only aspirin but also natural salicylates, which are found in many foods, especially fruits. He then began to suspect that there was one class of agent which cross-reacted with the salicylates, namely, the yellow food dye tetrazine, which can be fatal in patients who have an allergy to aspirin. He proceeded to take some of his patients off all yellow food dyes and found that not only their allergies but also their behavioral states improved. He subsequently tried this in children and reported rather remarkable changes in their hyperkinetic behavior.[33]

The trouble with the hypothesis is that it encompasses a whole range of substances. There are hundreds of artificial dyes and flavors (as well as preservatives) in foods, and many are low molecular weight substances which share the properties of tetrazine. This, according to Feingold, gives them their common action; although tetrazine is chemically unlike aspirin, it shares the low molecular weight property.

In a controlled experiment, a group of hyperkinetic children had red and yellow food dyes withdrawn from their diet.[34] In this kind of experiment, the parents inevitably think something great is going to happen. They have to go to a lot of fuss in preparing the food, and

*James Satterfield 1973: personal communication.

once they begin to focus on the child's symptoms and to invest a lot of effort, they begin to see things happening. The child suddenly becomes attended to, and a lot of his nonspecific symptoms disappear. For this reason, the control group consisted of another restricted diet—cottage cheese, cheeses, and egg products were withheld. The parents of both groups of children were told that the diets might or might not improve their child's behavior. The experiment was run double-blind and the groups crossed over. Among the first 10 patients on the experimental diet who were interviewed, 7 showed considerable improvement, and 3 of the parents reported that the child was as good or better on the diet than when receiving medication.[34]

A positive aspect of this study is that it clearly does no harm. One does not add anything to the diet but simply removes some things which probably should not have been there in the first place. (There is no reason, for example, that magarine has to be yellow. That so many foods are prepared with potentially harmful additives holds major implications for the food industry.) It is not necessarily recommended that one make parents go to all the effort, but the tetrazine-restricted diet is something that one may consider with a hyperkinetic child, especially if the parent finds that the child does not respond to drugs or is not willing to take them.

MISCELLANEOUS EXPERIMENTAL DRUG THERAPIES

Many of the most serious childhood psychiatric disorders continue to be refractory to available treatments, but there are a few things on the horizon. Campbell has studied triiodothyronine (T_3) in psychotic and in severely disturbed nonpsychotic children and found significant beneficial effects; both antipsychotic and stimulating actions have been seen in the treated children.[35] It is possible that we will see a return to the investigation of hormone treatments in severely disturbed children.

Recent attempts to reintroduce hydantoin compounds such as phenytoin (Dilantin) and anti-petit-mal drugs such as ethosuximide (Zarontin) for the treatment of learning and behavior disorders have not received much support. It was thought that phenytoin might be good for the impulsive, aggressive, acting-out child who may have a kind of subclinical epileptic picture. In a controlled trial, it was not effective for children with temper tantrums, although there had been some initial success in children presenting with severe tantrums.[2]

Cyproheptadine (Periactin) is a serotonin antagonist and an antihistamine which increases appetite and which may be useful in the treatment of anorexia nervosa, although the evidence for its efficacy is extremely limited. However, anorexia nervosa is a very serious disorder, and physicians treating adolescents with this problem may wish to consider a therapeutic trial of cyproheptadine.

REFERENCES

1. Eisenberg. L. and Conners, C.K.: Psychopharmacology in childhood. In Talbot, N.B., Kagan, J., and Eisenberg, L. (eds.): *Behavioral Science in Pediatric Medicine.* Philadelphia: W.B. Saunders Company, 1971.

2. Conners, C.K.: Organic therapies in child psychiatry. In Freedman, A.M., Kaplan, H.I., and Sadock, B.J. (eds.): *Comprehensive Textbook of Psychiatry.* 2d ed. Baltimore: The Williams & Wilkins Co., 1975, pp. 2240-2246.

3. Bender, L. and Nichtern, S.: Chemotherapy and child psychiatry. *NY State J. Med.* 56:2791-2795, 1956.

4. Freedman, A.M.: Drug therapy in behavior disorders. *Pediatr. Clin. North Am.* August, 1958, p. 573.

5. Freeman, R.D.: Drug effects on learning in children: a selective review of the past thirty years. *J. Spec. Ed.* 1:17, 1966.

6. Freeman, R.D.: Psychopharmacology and the retarded child. In Menolascino, F.J. (ed.): *Psychiatric Approaches to Mental Retardation in Childhood.* New York: Basic Books Inc., 1970.

7. Shader, R.I. and DiMascio, A.: *Psychotropic Drug Side Effects.* Baltimore: The Williams & Wilkins Co., 1970.

8. Fish, B., Shapiro, T., and Campbell, M.: Long-term prognosis and the response of schizophrenic children to drug therapy: a controlled study of trifluoperazine. *Am. J. Psychiatry* 123:32, 1966.

9. Engelhardt, D.M., Polizos, P., Waizer, J. et al: A double-blind comparison of fluphenazine and haloperidol. *J. Autism & Child. Schizophrenia* 3:128, 1973.

10. Engelhardt, D.M., Polizos, P., and Margolis, R.A.: The drug treatment of childhood psychosis. In Smith, W.L. (ed.): *Drugs, Development, and Cerebral Function.* Springfield, Ill: Charles C Thomas, 1972, pp. 224-234.

11. Tarsy, D. and Baldessarini, R.J.: The tardive dyskinesia syndrome. In Klawans, H.L. (ed.): *Clinical Neuropharmacology.* Vol. 1. New York: Raven Press, 1976.

12. McAndrew, J.B., Case, Q., and Treffert, D.: Effects of prolonged phenothiazine intake on psychotic and other hospitalized children. *J. Autism & Child. Schizophrenia* 2:75, 1972.

13. Waizer, J., Polizos, P., Hoffman, S.P. et al: A single-blind evaluation of thiothixene with outpatient schizophrenic children. *J. Autism & Child. Schizophrenia* 2:378, 1972.

14. Fish, B.: Treatment of children. In Kline, N.S. and Lehman, H.E. (eds.): *Psychopharmacology.* Boston: Little, Brown & Co., 1966.

15. Effron, A.S. and Freedman, A.M.: The treatment of behavior disorders in children with Benadryl. *J. Pediatr.* 42:261, 1953.

16. DiMascio. A.: The effects of benzodiazepines on aggression: reduced or increased? In Garattini, S., Mussini, E., and Randall, L.O. (eds.): *The Benzodiazepines.* New York: Raven Press, 1973, pp. 433-440.

17. Rapoport, J.L., Quinn, P.O., Bradbard, G. et al: Imipramine and methylphenidate treatment of hyperactive boys: a double-blind comparison. *Arch. Gen. Psychiatry* 30:789-793, 1974.

18. Frommer, E.A.: Treatment of childhood depression with anti-depressant drugs. *Br. Med. J.* 1:729-732, 1967.

19. Huessey, H.R. and Wright, A.: The use of imipramine in children's behavior disorders. *Acta Paedopsychiatr.* (Basel) 37:194, 1970.

20. Waizer, J., Hoffman, S.P., Polizos, P. et al: Outpatient treatment of hyperactive schoolchildren with imipramine. *Am. J. Psychiatry* 131:587, 1974.

21. Winsberg, B.G., Bailer, I., Kupietz, S. et al: Effects of imipramine and dextroamphetamine on the behavior of neuropsychiatrically impaired children. *Am. J. Psychiatry* 128:1425, 1972.

22. Kraepelin, E.: *Manic-Depressive Insanity and Paranoia.* Edinburgh: E. & S. Livingstone Ltd., 1921.

23. Kelly, J.T., Koch, M., and Bugel, D.: Lithium carbonate in juvenile manic-depressive illness. *Dis. Nerv. Sys.* 37:90-92, 1976.

24. Shader, R.I., Jackson, A.H., and Dodes, L.M.: The anti-aggressive effects of lithium in man. *Psychopharmacologia* 40:17-24, 1974.

25. Rifkin, A., Quitkin, F., Carillo, C. et al: Lithium carbonate in emotionally unstable character disorders. *Arch. Gen. Psychiatry* 27:519-523, 1972.

26. Conners, C.K. (ed.): *Clinical Use of Stimulant Drugs in Children.* The Hague: Excerpta Medica, 1974.

27. Millichap, J.G.: Drugs in the management of minimal brain dysfunction. *Ann. N.Y. Acad. Sci.* 205:321, 1973.

28. Satterfield, J.H.: EEG issues in children with minimal brain dysfunction. *Sem. Psychiatry* 5:35, 1973.

29. Conners, C.K., Taylor, E., Meo, G. et al: Magnesium pemoline and dextroamphetamine: a controlled study in children with minimal brain dysfunction. *Psychopharmacologia* 26:321, 1972.

30. Page, J.G., Bernstein, J.E., Janicki, R.S. et al: A multiclinic trial of pemoline in childhood hyperkinesis. In Conners, C.K. (ed.): *Clinical Use of Stimulant Drugs in Children.* The Hague: Excerpta Medica, 1974.

31. Safer, D.J. and Allen, R.P.: Side effects from long-term use of stimulants in children. In Gittelman-Klein, R. (ed.): *Recent Advances in Child Psychopharmacology.* New York: Human Sciences Press, 1975.

32. Safer, D. and Allen, R.: Factors influencing the suppressant effects of stimulant drugs on the growth of hyperactive children. *Pediatrics* 51:660, 1973.

33. Feingold, B.: *Why Your Child is Hyperactive.* New York: Random House, Inc., 1974.

34. Conners, C.K., Goyette, C.H., Southwick, D.A. et al: Food additives and hyperkinesis: a controlled double-blind experiment. *Pediatrics* 58:154-166, 1976.

35. Campbell, M., Fish, B., David, R. et al: Liothyronine treatment in psychotic and nonpsychotic children under 6 years. *Arch. Gen. Psychiatry* 29:602-608, 1973.

9 Overview of Clinical Psychopharmacology in Childhood Disorders

Rachel Gittelman-Klein, Ph.D.

In the pharmacologic treatment of childhood behavior disorders, the practitioner is faced with a tactical dilemma: should the treatment be determined by the presence of specific symptoms or behaviors—such as hyperactivity, anxiety, and temper tantrums, to name only a few—or should the therapeutic endeavor be targeted towards the amelioration of a constellation of symptoms which form a syndrome or diagnostic entity—such as a hyperkinetic reaction or schizophrenia, childhood type? In other words, do we treat traits or illnesses?

In adult psychiatry, there is growing evidence that predictive validity for drug effects is enhanced by the use of a diagnostic approach. Thus, the treatment of "anxiety" will follow different patterns depending on whether one is dealing with anxious schizophrenic, anxious depressive, or anxious phobic patients. The observed relationship between treatment outcome and diagnosis has given support to the use of diagnostic classification.

The remaining challenge is often to refine criteria to maximize the usefulness of diagnostic entities in the prediction of treatment response. The degree to which we are able to determine therapeutic strategies for a specific diagnosis is a function of our state of knowledge. The fact that much of adult psychopharmacologic therapeutics is still aimed at discrete symptoms reflects a failure to understand fully, so far, the phenomenology and the diagnostic significance of these symptoms.

The above issues are most pertinent in childhood psychiatric disorders and in their psychopharmacologic management. In some cases, chemotherapy is clearly indicated on the basis of the diagnostic group (eg, hyperkinetic disorder); in others, it is directed at symptoms of a particular diagnostic group (eg, hyperactivity among "psychotic" children); and in yet other instances, chemotherapy may be attempted for single-symptom removal (eg, temper tantrums). Consequently, the judicious use of medications in children requires consideration of the diagnostic process.

HYPERKINETIC DISORDER

Hyperkinesis, as such, is a symptom. Minimally brain-damaged, grossly brain-damaged, retarded, nonretarded, psychotic, and non-psychotic children and others may show this symptom. Fish has emphasized the fallacy of the notion of the hyperactive child, noting that there are several types of children who show hyperactive behavior with varying degrees of personality disorganization.[1] Yet in spite of the relatively wide distribution of the symptom across childhood disorders, there is little disagreement regarding the symptoms which characterize the diagnostic entities of hyperkinetic reactions of childhood. There is a consensus that children so diagnosed display, for their age, excessive motor activity, impulsivity, short attention span, low tolerance for frustration, and often, aggressivity—all in the absence of schizophrenic or other psychotic symptoms. The above symptoms are of long duration, and by the time a psychiatrist sees the child, difficulties are typically of long standing. The critical diagnostic issues in hyperkinesis are: (1) the number of these characteristics necessary for the diagnosis; (2) when and under what circumstances the symptoms have to be manifest; and (3) how early in the child's life the diagnosis can be made.

There are no clear-cut criteria for the diagnosis. Nor are there rules indicating which and how many of the traits justify the diagnosis. Further, the behavior of different children who share some or all of the traits is extremely variable, so that difficulties vary in intensity and across situations.[2] The status of the diagnosis of hyperkinetic children is indeed problematic, yet despair is not in order. Researchers in the field of psychopharmacology have been able to demonstrate very marked drug effects among children diagnosed as hyperkinetic, thereby indicating that even in this state of diagnostic uncertainty clear patterns of outcome can be discerned.

Central to the diagnosis is a report by teachers of the child's inability to stick to his work or of his difficulty in completing work. Parents rarely report hyperactivity per se; rather, they complain of lack of cooperation, of difficulty in following through on instructions, and of poor work habits. In addition, a history of such difficulties is extremely common. It is not unusual for the symptoms to be absent during office visits. The failure to observe directly the signs of the disorder do not preclude its presence. (It is to be understood that whenever reference is made to hyperactivity or hyperkinesis in the present discussion, it is indicative of the diagnosis *hyperkinetic reaction of childhood* as defined by the *Diagnostic and Statistical Manual of Mental Disorders*;[3] conclusions drawn from this patient group cannot be generalized to psychotic or severely impaired children who, as part of their total clinical picture, also present symptoms of hyperactivity.)

Stimulants

The psychostimulants are the treatment of choice for hyperkinetic children. When a good effect is obtained, the child is not only "better," but his behavior is indistinguishable from that of normal children.[4] In addition, a very large proportion of hyperkinetic children respond to stimulants. Therefore, the drugs have a broad, as well as potent, therapeutic impact.

Of all pediatric psychopharmacologic interventions, the therapeutic effect of stimulants on the syndrome of hyperkinesis in children is the best substantiated. Their short-term usefulness has been demonstrated in several controlled studies, and a critical perusal of the literature clearly points to the conclusion that the therapeutic value of stimulants has been established for the amelioration of gross motor hyperactivity and short attention span. The practitioner can choose among the stimulants methylphenidate (Ritalin), dextroamphetamine (Dexedrine), magnesium pemoline (Cylert), or deanol (Deaner).

The amphetamines were the first compounds used in the treatment of hyperkinetic children and may fairly be considered among the oldest psychotropic agents still in currency. In spite of the reports by Bradley in the 1930s and Laufer in the 1950s, it was not until the 1960s, with the work of Conners and his co-workers, that the scientific investigation of stimulant activity gained impetus.[5][6] About 20 years after the first reports of amphetamine effects, methylphenidate was also reported clinically useful in the management of hyperkinetic children.[7][8] Since the 1960s, several controlled studies have documented the usefulness of this drug for the treatment of hyperactive children.[9-11] In 1973 caffeine was reported to be effective as well,[12] but more recent, placebo-controlled studies have failed to demonstrate significant therapeutic advantages of caffeine over placebo, and we must conclude that it does not offer a clinical alternative in the management of hyperkinetic children.[13-15]

There are no clinical differences between methylphenidate and dextroamphetamine. Both are short acting in their effect and last from two to six hours. Dosage requirements vary widely. Dextroamphetamine dosage varies between 5 and 40 mg per day; methylphenidate dosage, between 10 and 80 mg per day. Their side effects are very similar, consisting typically of loss or reduction of appetite and delay in onset of sleep, and occur in about 30% of children treated with moderately high doses. More rarely, mood changes consisting of interpersonal sensitivity, or "touchiness," and a sad demeanor may occur. The latter side effects are most marked at the initiation of treatment and often diminish over time. In a child who responds well, the presence of the untoward effects should not lead to a premature termination of treatment. Rather, the child should be followed over several weeks; if there is no adaptation to the medication, dosage should be reduced and subsequently increased very gradually if clinically indicated. Our clinical observation is that side effects are less likely to occur if dosage is built up in small increments.

There is suggestive data that stimulants, especially dextroamphetamine, may have an inhibiting effect on growth.[16] Consequently, methylphenidate might be the drug of choice, since it may be less noxious in this regard; however, this is not established yet. A recent investigation failed to find a reduction in growth among early adolescents treated with stimulants in childhood.[17]

The data published on growth inhibition show a wide variation in the growth suppression effect. This variability indicates that it is only a subgroup of the total treated sample who are vulnerable to this side effect. Further, larger children seem more at risk than others. These results are reassuring to the extent that the growth of most of the children will probably not be affected deleteriously. Nevertheless, a growth chart should be kept on all children treated with stimulants so that the clinician might be alerted to the possible presence of growth inhibition. In such cases, dosage reduction, as well as drug holidays, should be considered. Drug holidays are often problematic for children on moderate to high doses since the abrupt cessation of the medication may cause a rebound effect during which their behavior is even worse than it was before treatment was begun.

Because of the stimulant properties of magnesium pemoline in adults, its efficacy in the treatment of hyperactive children was investigated in two well-designed studies.[18] [19] The major differences in the activity of this drug compared to that of other stimulants are its two- to three-week delay in inducing significant clinical effects, and its long-acting property. That magnesium pemoline can be administered in a single dose represents a distinct advantage over other stimulants. The necessity for midday doses presents practical and clinical problems. Supervision of medication ingestion in the schools is difficult. Even when easily arranged, the greater the number of daily administrations, the greater the opportunity for both regimen deviation and for singling out the child as different from his peers. Another important disadvantage of multiple doses is the marked increase in the likelihood of side effects such as anorexia and insomnia. Therefore, it seems that magnesium pemoline should be the first drug considered for the clinical management of hyperkinetic children, methylphenidate the second, and dextroamphetamine the third. In contrast to that of the other stimulants, the use of magnesium pemoline necessitates blood tests for liver function at regular intervals since there may be an elevation in SGOT values reported. The abnormality may not be sustained and its significance is unclear. Discontinuation should be considered if the pathologic findings are consistent over time.

Length of therapy The question arises as to how long stimulants can be used in hyperkinetic children. It used to be thought that the disorder reflected a maturational lag and did not linger beyond puberty. Hence, treatment was limited to middle childhood. Though the symptom of hyperactivity diminishes markedly with age, attentional and social handicaps frequently remain through adolescence.[11] [20] Clinical evidence is accumulating which suggests that stimulants continue to exert a positive effect, without concurrent euphoria, in grown-up hyperkinetic children with residual symptomatology. Our own clinical experience in treating children into adolescence is consonant with this observation. The risk for amphetamine abuse has been invoked to argue against the use of stimulants at any age level; however, all data available so far have failed to reveal an increased prevalence of drug abuse in youngsters treated with stimulants. This already remote danger is even further reduced—perhaps eliminated—with the use of magnesium pemoline, which does not have euphoriant effects at therapeutic dose levels, and which therefore would not trigger a possible vicious cycle of positive mood effect, tolerance, increased intake, and so on which might evolve into an addictive pattern.

Phenothiazines

Total refractoriness to stimulant treatment is extremely rare (about 10% or less) but may occur. In some instances there may be intolerance to the stimulants. In such cases, other therapeutic options exist. The child may be treated with phenothiazines or tricyclics.

The effects of the phenothiazines are not as well documented as are those of the stimulants. One study failed to observe improvement differences between prochlorperazine and placebo in hyperactive children.[21] In contrast, significant therapeutic effects have been found with chlorpromazine and thioridazine.[10] [22-24] Phenothiazines are as effective as stimulants in reducing the level of motor activity in hyperactive children. The range of improvement, however, is broader with stimulants than it is with phenothiazines, which, while they reduce motor activity, do not affect other behaviors as markedly as do the stimulants.

Dosages of up to 200 mg of thioridazine or chlorpromazine are necessary. Beyond this level, no clinical advantage is accrued and side effects increase considerably. The side effects associated with phenothiazine treatment in children are very different from those associated with treatment with stimulants. Drowsiness and weight gain are typical. Enuresis (usually nocturnal, very occasionally diurnal as well) may occur with use of thioridazine.

Tricyclics

Imipramine has been demonstrated to improve the behavior of hyperkinetic children,[25] [26] and it offers certain practical advantages in that it is long acting and thus eliminates or reduces the need for multiple doses throughout the day. Further, clinical side effects are reported to be negligible. However, as with the phenothiazines, the effect of imipramine is not as complete as with stimulants and many children fail to sustain their initially good response.[27] Also, the potential usefulness of high dosage of this drug has been limited by recent reports of cardiotoxic electrocardiographic effects in children.[28] [29]

Many studies have used heterogeneous groups of children with a variety of behavior problems and learning problems. That hyperactivity is regularly reduced by pharmacologic treatment in spite of the sample heterogeneity attests to the real value of medications in this disorder. At the same time, it is also conceivable that the stimulants have a broader spectrum of action and could play a useful role in the treatment of other childhood behavior disorders. So far, this issue has not been studied systematically, and the only valid conclusion which may be drawn from the empirical findings available is that the stimulants have an unequivocal value in the treatment of the hyperkinetic syndrome. Indications for other conditions, such as nonspecific behavior disorders, remain unproven.

Nontreatment Factors Influencing Drug Response

Empirical findings in regard to the contention that medications have a selective effect on brain-damaged hyperactive children are ambiguous.[30] Satterfield et al have reported greater improvement with drug treatment in those children with minimal brain dysfunction who show both electroencephalographic and neurologic abnormalities than in those children with minimal brain dysfunction who show neither of these abnormalities.[31] However, the proportions of children who improved in each group did not differ statistically. Further, it is conceivable that children with both electroencephalographic and neurologic abnormalities were more behaviorally disturbed, so that the difference in degree of improvement might reflect differences in symptomatology. Since the children were not selected for hyperactivity, it is not known how many were hyperactive, and therefore the validity of generalizing the findings is problematic.

A similar problem exists in a study on dextroamphetamine which reports a relationship between clinical neurologic signs and treatment response.[32] The actual contribution of organicity to outcome remains unclear since there was a positive relationship between organicity and initial level of hyperkinesis.

In sum, there is accumulating, but not conclusive, evidence that neurologic dysfunction plays a role in mediating the response of hyperkinetic children to stimulants. The clinical lesson to be derived from the studies seems to be that neurologically impaired children with a less than clear-cut pattern of hyperkinesis should be given a trial of stimulant administration. On the other hand, no child who displays the symptoms of a hyperkinetic reaction, even without neurologic signs, should be deprived of the opportunity to receive a trial of stimulant treatment.

In addition to the role of brain dysfunction in mediating drug response, the relationship of clinical improvement to other physiologic characteristics, such as skin resistance and central nervous system evoked potentials, has been examined.[33-36] The work has considerable theoretical importance but little clinical significance, and there is no reason to recommend that physicians obtain these technologically difficult measures.

Aspects of psychopathology not related to diagnosis, such as severity or stability of symptoms, do not discriminate between responders and nonresponders. Environmental factors, such as quality of home and mother-child relationship, have also failed to relate to drug therapy outcome.[23] [24]

There is a disproportionate number of boys among hyperkinetic youngsters, but sex has not been found to be associated with improvement. On the other hand, young, preschool hyperactive children show a more variable response to the stimulants. The lack of drug effect in a large proportion of very young children as compared to older ones may reflect greater diagnostic ambiguity, and therefore diagnostic inaccuracy, among the younger group.[37] [38] At the same time, it is conceivable that there is an age-related physiologic variability which affects drug response.

In summary, it appears brain dysfunction and level of physiologic reactivity may be relevant dimensions in the prediction of drug effects among hyperactive children, but these factors are of no significance for clinical management. Much controversy surrounds the use of medications for the management of behavior disorders in children. Behavior therapy has been suggested as an effective alternative to drugs; indeed, some investigators have demonstrated the clinical efficacy of behavioral techniques in hyperactive children. In a study comparing the effects of behavior modification techniques to those of methylphenidate, both treatments were found to be helpful, but the therapeutic impact of methylphenidate was significantly superior to that of behavior therapy. Therefore, though the behavioral techniques are useful, they are not the most effective interventions in hyperkinetic children.[4]

ANXIETY DISORDERS

Severely disturbed, psychotic children, who often display anxious mood and behavior, are excluded from consideration here. There are other children who experience marked anxiety in the absence of gross deviations in personality or cognitive development. The youngsters may be tense, apprehensive, or overly concerned about performance in social or achievement-oriented situations. To this extent the children resemble adults with anxiety symptoms and obsessional traits. Children typically do not display motor agitation, a symptom often interpreted (though questionably so) as an anxiety symptom in adult psychopathology.

The treatment of anxiety disorders in children is quite different from that in adults. The role of the minor tranquilizers, such as diazepam (Valium) and chlordiazepoxide (Librium), has not been explored. Low doses of phenothiazines are used in many clinical settings, but their efficacy is undocumented and their prescription remains a matter of individual, empirical practice. Small doses (25 mg of chlorpromazine or thioridazine) are not usually associated with troublesome side effects, but susceptibility to side effects is very variable, and it is possible for drowsiness to occur with low doses of the phenothiazines.

Separation anxiety is the one type of anxiety in children which is exquisitely amenable to pharmacotherapy. In moderation, this anxiety is not pathologic, but it may become so severe that the child experiences marked difficulties separating from the mother. Such children become dysfunctional. In the extreme, they cannot attend school or participate in any activity—such as visiting friends, going shopping, or going to camp—which calls for separation.

The genesis of pathologic separation anxiety is very different from that of most of the other childhood disorders, which tend to be chronic. In contrast, separation anxiety comes on quite suddenly, in a matter of a few weeks, in children whose adjustment was previously unremarkable. In about 80% of the cases, it follows a change in the child's environment, such as a move or school change, or illness or loss of a relative. Further, the disorder tends to be self-limiting, and spontaneous remissions occur regularly. Nevertheless, in some instances the affected period may be extended and last for years. The disorder occurs equally often in boys and girls. The clinical syndrome has been described widely: children with the disorder experience anxiety to the point of panic when separation is attempted. They are plagued with morbid fears and worries concerning their parents' welfare, or sometimes their own. They tend to be clinging, demanding children. During the acute phase of the illness, they are extremely manipulative and may become incensed, even aggressive, if they are forced into situations which make them anxious. The anxiety often has marked diurnal fluctuations, worsening in the morning and evening. Psychophysiologic symptoms are common and usually consist of stomachaches, nausea, or vague aches and pains.

Children with severe separation anxiety are often described as depressed.[39] They do not, however, exhibit the anhedonia or the pessimism typical of adult depressives. The sad look they regularly present when seen professionally can be viewed as being a reaction to being confronted with their difficulties. When no demands or threats of separation are made, the children can enjoy themselves easily. Therefore, it is felt that it is diagnostically erroneous to consider pathologic separation anxiety the equivalent of adult depressive disorder.

Some argue that the onset of this disorder in adolescence is a harbinger of severe pathology such as schizophrenia. We have found no evidence for this clinical claim. The age of onset does not appear to be associated with a differential natural outcome or with drug response.

Imipramine effects are very marked among children and adolescents with severe separation anxiety. In some cases the effect is noticeable within as little as a week. Most children require three to four weeks of treatment before symptom amelioration clearly occurs. Good clinical results are very dramatic; the child becomes totally free of morbid preoccupations. However, he still retains the conviction that his previous worries will return to plague him, and he will continue to resist separation. Therefore, the pharmacologic treatment of this childhood disorder regularly needs to be combined with a vigorous therapeutic effort aimed at reducing anticipatory anxiety and increasing the child's independence. This aspect of treatment is detailed further in a recent publication.[40]

Dosages of up to 150 mg per day are typically necessary. Side effects are not usually troublesome; the most common are dry mouth and constipation, which occur in about 50% and 30%, respectively, of the children treated with doses of 75 to 175 mg per day.[41] Cardiotoxic effects, consisting of T wave change, PR interval lengthening, and QRS broadening, are of concern in this group since relatively high dosages may be required. However, these changes are not associated with abnormal clinical findings, and therefore their substantive significance remains obscure. A recommendation has been made by the Food and Drug Administration that imipramine dosage in children not exceed 5 mg/kg per day.

Many patients treated with imipramine require six to eight weeks of treatment to attain clinical amelioration. Following this crucial period, imipramine dosage can usually be lowered to a maintenance level approximately half that of the maximum therapeutic dose. Further, if a patient has not responded to imipramine at higher doses within six to eight weeks, it is quite unlikely that he will respond to continued imipramine treatment. Therefore, it is the first two months of treatment that should evoke concern regarding cardiac changes.

On the basis of the data obtained, baseline electrocardiograms should be obtained for those children to be treated with imipramine in dosages approximating 3.5 to 5.0 mg/kg daily. The vast majority of children treated for enuresis with smaller imipramine doses would be excluded from this consideration, but those treated for school phobia or hyperkinesis would not. After there is clinical amelioration, imipramine dosage should be decreased to a level that is consonant with maintenance of gains. Only in children whose daily long-term maintenance dosage of imipramine is 3.5 mg/kg or more does electrocardiographic monitoring every two months seem desirable.

The use of imipramine in children with severe separation anxiety can be of relatively short duration, and in this regard it stands out as an exception to general psychopharmacologic practice. In most cases administration of imipramine need not be long-term, and frequently children remain symptom-free after a three- to four-month treatment period. Since children are susceptible to withdrawal symptoms from imipramine (nausea, stomachache), the dosage should be reduced gradually over a two-week period.

DEPRESSIVE DISORDERS

The presence of well-defined depressive disorders in children is not well documented. There is little question that unhappy, miserable children are numerous. Whether their dysphoric mood reflects a reaction to an unrewarding environment or a primary mood disorder is problematic. In spite of a few studies in the area, there is no adequate documentation of the therapeutic merits of antidepressants in children deemed to be depressive by means of well-defined clinical criteria.[42] The data suggest that mechanisms of mood regulation differ between children and adults.[43]

Attempts to identify children with clear-cut depressive symptomatology are underway. Using the adult Research Diagnostic Criteria for depression,[44] Puig-Antich, in a pilot study, has identified a number of inpatient children as depressed and has also reported clear imipramine effects in such youngsters.* This recent, ongoing investigation represents one of the first attempts at using in children those diagnostic criteria which are known to be useful for identifying depressive disorders in adults. It is possible that reviews of clinical psychopharmacology in the future will legitimately include a discussion of the treatment of childhood depression, and that the latter will have evolved as a well-defined clinical entity.

---

*J. Puig-Antich 1976: personal communication.

CHILDHOOD PSYCHOSIS

An array of behavioral syndromes is included under the diagnostic umbrella of childhood psychosis. The current official nomenclature does not distinguish among the various disorders, and all are lumped under the rubric of schizophrenia, childhood type. There is agreement among workers in the field that age of onset is an important classificatory characteristic. Consequently, the diagnosis *early infantile autism* is used for disorders in children in whom onset is in the first two to three years of life; those disorders of somewhat later onset have been called *disintegrative psychoses*, or *early childhood psychoses*. Children in these two groups are markedly different in overt symptomatology from young adult schizophrenics. The vast majority of the children are intellectually retarded and do not present Bleulerian symptoms. Rather, they are socially withdrawn, have bizarre interests and deviant language development, and often have marked mood lability. There is a debate as to whether these childhood clinical states represent early forms of adult schizophrenia or distinct pathologic entities.

It is not possible to estimate the role of antipsychotic medication in childhood psychosis from the known effects of this class of drugs in adult schizophrenia. These childhood disorders represent an instance in which the diagnostic approach is not helpful for pharmacotherapy, except in a negative fashion. That is, a diagnosis of childhood psychosis will not indicate what drugs to use, but rather what drugs to avoid. Stimulants tend to worsen the condition of severely disturbed youngsters (and in this respect the latter resemble adult schizophrenics), and therefore the use of stimulants is contraindicated in psychotic children.

Neuroleptics can be extremely helpful in ameliorating secondary symptoms such as hyperactivity, aggressivity, mood lability, lack of appetite, and sleep difficulties, but they do not have a "normalizing" effect on the behavior of psychotic children. They do not modify positively the behavior of hypoactive, apathetic, anergic psychotic children, who are more like "burnt-out" chronic schizophrenics. They may, however, render an uncontrollable, disruptive psychotic youngster more manageable, and such an effect should not be denigrated. Some hyperactive or aggressive psychotic children can wreak havoc in a family. With the use of neuroleptics, institutionalization often can be avoided and school attendance becomes a possibility. However, in no case do the children become symptom-free. The disorder's cardinal symptoms of impaired social and communicative functions persist despite treatment, and the child's adjustment continues to be markedly impaired.

Diphenhydramine has been recommended as a safe, often effective drug in psychoses of early childhood. However, consistent objective evidence of this drug's efficacy is lacking. In a three-month, placebo-controlled study of diphenhydramine vs chlorpromazine in psychotic children, diphenhydramine, in doses of about 800 mg per day, was no better than placebo and caused considerable side effects.* In contrast, chlorpromazine was significantly superior to the other two treatments for a number of secondary symptoms.

Neuroleptics tend to be tolerated better by psychotic children than by children with other psychiatric disorders. Dosages range up to 500 mg for chlorpromazine or thioridazine, 15 to 20 mg for haloperidol or fluphenazine, and 45 mg for thiothixene. The most common clinical side effects are drowsiness and weight gain.

Recently, neuroleptic withdrawal has been found to be associated with neurologic symptoms in psychotic children. The phenomenon is reminiscent of the tardive dyskinesias which are being reported with increasing frequency among adult patients treated with neuroleptics.[45] Involuntary movements appear within 1 to 15 days after withdrawal of the drug. In 50% of the cases, the symptoms remit spontaneously within one to two weeks, and they are regularly reversible with reinstitution of treatment. These movements, though similar to adult dyskinesias, differ from the latter in that they do not typically involve the buccolingual area, but rather the arms, trunk, and head. Their incidence is related to total dose exposure and length of treatment.[46] Drugs seem to vary in their contributions to neurologic withdrawal symptoms, which are more likely to occur with the use of high-potency neuroleptics such as fluphenazine or thiothixene (50% to 80% of cases) than with the low-potency ones such as chlorprothixene or thioridazine (10% to 30%).[47]

Because of these symptoms, the ultimate significance of which is unknown, drug holidays are strongly recommended—in all cases where this is at all feasible—for children whose severe psychopathology necessitates long-term neuroleptic treatment.

CONDUCT DISORDERS

Antisocial, delinquent behavior patterns represent a serious challenge to attempts at effective treatment. Neither methylphenidate nor diphenylhydantoin has been effective in inducing behavioral improvement in inpatient boys below the age of 15.[48] In contrast, dextroamphetamine, in dosages of up to 40 mg per day, was found to

---

*D.M. Engelhardt 1976: personal communication.

be superior to placebo in reducing aggressivity and in improving sociability in antisocial male outpatients of 13 to 18 years of age. Interestingly, the most improved youngsters were the ones who had been rated before treatment as more hyperactive.[49] These results would seem to suggest a relationship between early hyperkinesis and later, adolescent conduct disorders. On the other hand, the clinical improvement recorded might be due to a nonspecific, amphetamine-induced mood elevation which in turn may have led to a diminution of antisocial behavior. The efficacy of psychostimulants in aggressive, delinquent youngsters remains questionable. In addition, the serious danger of abuse, especially great in this group, cannot be minimized. Magnesium pemoline offers a real advantage in this respect, since it is not believed to have an addictive potential as great as that of dextroamphetamine or methylphenidate.

Violent temper outbursts, a narrow aspect of conduct disorders, have been treated with diphenylhydantoin and placebo with no appreciable treatment differences observed. This drug appears to have no value in episodic, sudden, violent outbursts, although a response was expected, as this symptom characteristic was thought to be possibly related to a type of central nervous system disorder which might respond to an anticonvulsant.[50]

GENERAL CLINICAL CONSIDERATIONS

Certain practices which are extremely helpful, yet often neglected, in the pharmacologic treatment of childhood disorders deserve mention. For example, sources of information regarding a child's response to treatment should not be limited to the parents; the school should always be consulted if the child's symptoms are manifest in the classroom setting as well as at home. In some cases, even if there are no complaints from school, teachers should be queried to ascertain that side effects such as drowsiness are not interfering with the child's academic performance. Input from the school is also often helpful in formulating a diagnosis.

Dosage levels are very variable, and there are no guidelines (such as age, weight, or body surface) to indicate a specific dosage range. Therefore, a flexible approach is necessary. If a child who has obtained good results with a drug deteriorates, it should not be assumed that the medication is no longer effective. Often, increments in dosage will reestablish a positive response. Children on medication should be followed on a regular basis to evaluate their status as regards side effects and continued need for drug treatment (many children who have been prescribed low dosages of medication are kept on these for extended periods of time and are never examined again). Also, children should be given "off-drug" periods, or "drug holidays," on a regular basis to determine the ongoing clinical usefulness of the drug and to minimize whatever deleterious effects might potentially be associated with the medication.

Parents should never be left to regulate dosage or to make decisions to terminate or continue treatment. Parents may overreact to minor or temporary changes in behavior; they may underestimate the degree of the child's difficulty; or, finally, they may use the medication in a punitive fashion. Therefore, medication adjustments should reflect a consensus between the family and the physician.

Finally, it is unusual for medication to be the sole intervention necessary (except in some cases of hyperkinesis where stimulants completely eliminate symptoms and where the parent-child relationships are good). Therefore, medication can rarely be viewed as a total treatment in children with behavior disorders.

This summary of childhood psychopharmacology obviously is not exhaustive. Campbell has reviewed the effects of drugs in childhood psychosis.[51] A more comprehensive guide to clinical management of the hyperkinetic syndrome has been presented by Katz et al, and the research literature on treatment of hyperkinesis up to 1974 has been reviewed critically.[52][53] Conners and Rapoport have presented lucid discussions of diagnosis and treatment of depression in children.[43][54] Consultation of these reviews is recommended for further information.

REFERENCES

1. Fish, B.: The 'one child, one drug' myth of stimulants in hyperkinesis. Importance of diagnostic categories in evaluating treatment. *Arch. Gen. Psychiatry* 25:193-203, 1971.

2. Klein, D.F. and Gittelman-Klein, R.: Problems in the diagnosis of minimal brain dysfunction and the hyperkinetic syndrome. In Gittelman-Klein, R. (ed.): *Recent Advances in Child Psychopharmacology*. New York: Human Sciences Press, 1975, pp. 47-63.

3. American Psychiatric Association: *Diagnostic and Statistical Manual of Mental Disorders*. 2d ed. Washington, D.C: American Psychiatric Association, 1968.

4. Gittelman-Klein, R. et al: Relative efficacy of methylphenidate and behavior modification in hyperkinetic children: an interim report. *J. Abnorm. Child Psychol.* 4:361-379, 1976.

5. Conners, C.K.: The effect of Dexedrine on rapid discrimination and motor control of hyperkinetic children under mild stress. *J. Nerv. & Ment. Dis.* 142:429-433, 1966.

6. Conners, C.K., Eisenberg, L., and Barcai, A.: Effect of dextroamphetamine on children. *Arch. Gen. Psychiatry* 17:478-485, 1967.

7. Knobel, M.: Psychopharmacology for the hyperkinetic child. *Arch. Gen. Psychiatry* 6:198, 1962.

8. Knobel, M. and Lytton, G.J.: Diagnosis and treatment of behavior disorders in children. *Dis. Nerv. Sys.* 20:334-340, 1958.

9. Conners, C.K. and Eisenberg, L.: The effects of methylphenidate on symptomatology and learning in disturbed children. *Am. J. Psychiatry* 120:458-464, 1963.

10. Gittelman-Klein, R., Klein, D.F., Katz, S. et al: Comparative effects of methylphenidate and thioridazine in hyperkinetic children. *Arch. Gen. Psychiatry* 33:1217-1231, 1976.

11. Weiss, G., Minde, K., Douglas, V. et al: Comparison of the effects of chlorpromazine, dextroamphetamine and methylphenidate on the behavior and intellectual functioning of hyperactive children. *Can. Med. J.* 104:20-25, 1971.

12. Schnackenburg, R.C.: Caffeine as a substitute for Schedule II stimulants in hyperkinetic children. *Am. J. Psychiatry* 130:796-800, 1973.

13. Conners, C.K.: A placebo-crossover study of caffeine treatment of hyperkinetic children. In Gittelman-Klein, R. (ed.): *Recent Advances in Child Psychopharmacology.* New York: Human Sciences Press, 1975, pp. 136-147.

14. Garfinkel, B.D., Webster, C.D., and Sloman, L.: Methylphenidate and caffeine in the treatment of children with minimal brain dysfunction. *Am. J. Psychiatry* 132:723, 1975.

15. Huestis, R.D., Arnold, L.E. and Smeltzer, D.J.: Caffeine vs methylphenidate and dextroamphetamine in minimal brain dysfunction: a double-blind comparison. *Am. J. Psychiatry* 132:868-871, 1975.

16. Safer, D.J. and Allen, R.P.: Side effects from long-term use of stimulants in children. In Gittelman-Klein, R. (ed.): *Recent Advances in Child Psychopharmacology.* New York: Human Sciences Press, 1975, pp. 109-122.

17. Gross, M.D.: Growth of hyperkinetic children taking methylphenidate, dextroamphetamine, or imipramine/desipramine. *Pediatrics* 58:423-431, 1976.

18. Conners, C.K., Taylor, E., Meo, G. et al: Magnesium pemoline and dextroamphetamine: a controlled study in children with minimal brain dysfunction. *Psychopharmacologia* 26:321-336, 1972.

19. Page, J.G., Bernstein, J.E., Janicki, R.S. et al: A multi-clinic trial of pemoline in childhood hyperkinesis. In Conners, C.K. (ed.): *Clinical Use of Stimulant Drugs in Children.* The Hague: Excerpta Medica, 1974, pp. 98-124.

20. Minde, K., Weiss, G., and Mendelson, N.: A five-year follow-up study of 91 hyperactive school children. *J. Am. Acad. Child Psychiatry* 11:595, 1972.

21. Cytryn, L., Gilbert, L., and Eisenberg, L.: The effectiveness of tranquilizing drugs plus supportive psychotherapy in treating behavior disorders of children: a double-blind study of 80 outpatients. *Am. J. Orthopsychiatry* 30:113-129, 1960.

22. Greenberg, L.M., Deem, M.A., and McMahon, S.: Effects of dextroamphetamine, chlorpromazine and hydroxyzine on behavior and performance in hyperactive children. *Am. J. Psychiatry* 129:532-539, 1972.

23. Weiss, G., Werry, J., Minde, K. et al: Studies on the hyperactive child. V. The effects of dextroamphetamine and chlorpromazine on behavior and intellectual functioning. *J. Child Psychol. Psychiatry* 9:145-156, 1968.

24. Werry, J.S., Weiss, G., Douglas, V. et al: Studies on the hyperactive child. III. The effect of chlorpromazine upon behavior and learning ability. *J. Am. Acad. Child Psychiatry* 5:292-312, 1966.

25. Greenberg, L.M., Yellin, A.M., Spring, C. et al: Clinical effects of imipramine and methylphenidate in hyperactive children. In Gittelman-Klein, R. (ed.): *Recent Advances in Child Psychopharmacology*. New York: Human Sciences Press, 1975, pp. 148-159.

26. Rapoport, J.L., Quinn, P.O., Bradbard, G. et al: Imipramine and methylphenidate treatments of hyperactive boys: a double-blind comparison. *Arch. Gen. Psychiatry* 30:789-793, 1974.

27. Gittelman-Klein, R.: Pilot clinical trial of imipramine in hyperkinetic children. In Conners, C.K. (ed.): *Clinical Use of Stimulant Drugs in Children*. The Hague: Excerpta Medica, 1974, pp. 192 201.

28. Saraf, K.R., Klein, D.F., Gittelman-Klein, R. et al: EKG effects of imipramine treatment in children. *J. Acad. Child Psychiatry*, in press.

29. Winsberg, B.G., Goldstein, S., Yepe, L.E. et al: Imipramine and electrocardiographic abnormalities in hyperactive children. *Am. J. Psychiatry* 132:542-545, 1975.

30. Laufer, M.W. and Denhoff, E.: Hyperkinetic behavior syndrome in children. *J. Pediatrics* 50:463-474, 1957.

31. Satterfield, J.H., Lesser, L.I., Saul, R.E. et al: EEG aspects in the diagnosis and treatment of minimal brain dysfunction. *Ann. N.Y. Acad. Sci.* 205:274-282, 1973.

32. Steinberg, G.S., Troshinsky, C., and Steinberg, H.C.: Dextro-amphetamine-responsive behavior disorder in schoolchildren. *Am. J. Psychiatry* 128:174-179, 1971.

33. Buchsbaum, M. and Wender, P.: Average evoked responses in normal and minimally brain dysfunctioned children treated with amphetamine. A preliminary report. *Arch. Gen. Psychiatry* 29:762-770, 1973.

34. Halliday, R., Rosenthal, J.H., Naylor, H. et al: Average evoked potential predictors of clinical improvement in hyperactive children treated with methylphenidate: an initial study and replication. *Psychophysiology* 13:429-440, 1976.

35. Prichep, L.S., Sutton, S., and Hakerem, G.: Evoked potentials in hyperkinetic and normal children under certainty and uncertainty: a placebo and methylphenidate study. *Psychophysiology* 13:419-428, 1976.

36. Satterfield, J.H., Cantwell, D.P., Lesser, L.I. et al: Physiological studies of the hyperkinetic child. I. *Am. J. Psychiatry* 128:102-108, 1972.

37. Conners, C.K.: Controlled trial of methylphenidate in preschool children with minimal brain dysfunction. In Gittelman-Klein, R. (ed.): *Recent Advances in Child Psychopharmacology*. New York: Human Sciences Press, 1975, pp. 64-78.

38. Schleifer, M., Weiss, G., Cohen, N. et al: Hyperactivity in pre-schoolers and the effect of methylphenidate. *Am. J. Orthopsychiatry* 45:38-50, 1975.

39. Frommer, E.A.: Treatment of childhood depression with anti-depressant drugs. *Br. Med. J.* 1:729-732, 1967.

40. Gittelman-Klein, R.: Pharmacotherapy and management of pathological separation anxiety. In Gittelman-Klein, R. (ed.): *Recent Advances in Child Psychopharmacology*. New York: Human Sciences Press, 1975, pp. 255-272.

41. Gittelman-Klein, R. and Klein, D.F.: School phobia: diagnostic considerations in the light of imipramine effects. *J. Nerv. & Ment. Dis.* 156:199-215, 1973.

42. Gittelman-Klein, R.: Definitional and methodological issues concerning depressive illness in children. In Schulterbrandt, J. and Raskin, A. (eds.): *Depression in Children: Conceptual Models, Diagnosis, and Treatment.* Washington, D.C: Government Printing Office, forthcoming.

43. Rapoport, J.L.: Psychopharmacology of childhood depression. In Klein, D.F. and Gittelman-Klein, R. (eds.): *Progress in Psychiatric Drug Treatment.* New York: Brunner/Mazel, Inc., 1976, pp. 493-505.

44. Spitzer, R.L., Endicott, J., and Robins, E.: Research Diagnostic Criteria (RDC). *Psychopharmacol. Bull.* 11:22-24, 1975.

45. Polizos, P., Engelhardt, D.M., Hoffman, S.P. et al: Neurological consequences of psychotropic drug withdrawal in schizophrenic children. *J. Autism & Child. Schizophrenia* 3:247-253, 1973.

46. McAndrew, J.B., Case, Q., and Treffert, D.A.: Effects of prolonged phenothiazine intake on psychotic and other hospitalized children. *J. Autism & Child. Schizophrenia* 2:75-91, 1972.

47. Engelhardt, D.M.: Neurological consequences of neuroleptic treatment of autistic children. Paper read before the 99th annual meeting of the American Association on Mental Deficiency, Portland, Oregon, May 19, 1975.

48. Conners, C.K., Kramer, R., Rothschild, G.H. et al: Treatment of young delinquent boys with diphenylhydantoin sodium and methylphenidate. *Arch. Gen. Psychiatry* 24:156-160, 1971.

49. Maletzky, B.M.: Dextroamphetamine and delinquency: hyperkinesis persisting? *Dis. Nerv. Sys.* 35:543-547, 1974.

50. Looker, A. and Conners, C.K.: Diphenylhydantoin in children with severe temper tantrums. *Arch. Gen. Psychiatry* 23:80-89, 1970.

51. Campbell, M.: Pharmacotherapy in early infantile autism. *Biol. Psychiat.* 10:399-423, 1975.

52. Katz, S., Saraf, K., Gittelman-Klein, R. et al: Clinical pharmacological management of hyperkinetic children. *Int. J. Ment. Hlth.* 4:157-181, 1975.

53. Gittelman-Klein, R.: Review of clinical treatment of hyperkinesis. In Klein, D.F. and Gittelman-Klein, R. (eds.): *Progress in Psychiatric Drug Treatment.* New York: Brunner/Mazel, Inc., 1975, pp. 661-674.

54. Conners, C.K.: Classification and treatment of childhood depression and depressive equivalents. In Gallant, D.M. and Simpson, G.M. (eds.): *Depression: Behavioral, Diagnostic, and Treatment Concepts.* New York: Spectrum Publications, Inc., 1976, pp. 181-204.

10 Medical Aspects of Psychotropic Drugs

Jerrold G. Bernstein, M.D.

INTRODUCTION

Effective prescription of psychotropic drugs for psychiatric illness must recognize that, in addition to their behavioral effects, these compounds are also likely to have rather widespread and complex effects on body physiology and chemistry. These medical consequences derive from three basic sources. First, the drugs themselves may produce side effects which may be either idiosyncratic or specifically related to their pharmacology. Second, psychotropic drugs may produce physiologic changes which may affect an existing medical condition in the patient. Third, these drugs may interact with other medications the patient may be taking. Therefore, a thorough understanding of the pharmacology of the psychotropic drugs is essential to their effective use and is also of prime importance in avoiding unpleasant, and at times dangerous, medical consequences of this form of psychiatric treatment.

From a clinical standpoint, psychotropic drugs are most usefully classified according to their primary effects: antipsychotic, antianxiety, antidepressant, and mood-stabilizing (see Table 1, p. 41). For the most part, discussion will focus on medical aspects of antipsychotic and antidepressant drugs and lithium; allusion will also be made to psychiatric aspects of certain medical drugs.

PERIPHERAL EFFECTS OF ANTIPSYCHOTIC DRUGS AND THEIR MANAGEMENT

The antipsychotic drugs may be divided into five groups according to their chemical structures: phenothiazines, butyrophenones, thioxanthenes, dihydroindolones, and dibenzoxazepines (see Table 1, p. 41).[1] The phenothiazine and butyrophenone antipsychotic drugs are the ones most widely used clinically. For practical purposes, the thioxanthene drugs are quite similar to the phenothiazines in their spectrum of activity and side effects. Because of the newness of the dihydroindolone and dibenzoxazepine antipsychotic drugs, there is not sufficient data to discuss them at length.

Antiadrenergic Effects

All known antipsychotic drugs have been shown to be capable of blocking the action of dopamine, a neurotransmitter substance in the brain. It is generally believed that the antipsychotic action of these drugs relates to this pharmacologic property. Further, there is a correlation between antipsychotic and dopamine-blocking potencies.[2][3] For example, chlorpromazine (Thorazine), which is among the weaker antipsychotic drugs, is also among the weaker dopamine blockers, while haloperidol (Haldol), one of the most potent antipsychotic drugs, has an exceedingly high affinity for dopamine receptors.[4]

The antipsychotic drugs also produce alpha-adrenergic blockade in the peripheral vascular system.[1][5] This effect is not generally desirable, as it may lead to a significant fall in blood pressure which can result in fainting or falling. Chlorpromazine and thioridazine (Mellaril) are the most potent in this regard and are therefore most likely to produce postural hypotension and fainting. Trifluoperazine (Stelazine) and fluphenazine (Prolixin) are less hypotensive, and haloperidol is the least likely to produce a fall in blood pressure, even at quite high therapeutic doses.[5][6] Of significance in this regard, however, is the fact that the phenothiazines (particularly chlorpromazine), when administered intramuscularly with haloperidol (also intramuscularly), may make the patient particularly susceptible to a hypotensive response.* Clinicians must understand the hypotensive potential of the antipsychotic drugs and attempt to guard against it by using them cautiously—particularly in elderly patients, patients with cardiovascular disease, and other patients who might be especially vulnerable to hypotension. In such patients, haloperidol is probably the safest antipsychotic drug to use. It is also important to begin antipsychotic drug therapy with relatively small dosages divided throughout the day, until the patient's response to the drug is known. At this point therapy may be converted to a single daily dose, generally best given at bedtime.

Some antipsychotic drugs may also produce electrocardiographic changes.[6][7] The changes generally observed are a flattening of the T wave, or ST segment changes that may resemble those abnormalities seen with ischemic coronary heart disease. Thioridazine and chlorpromazine are more likely to produce such electrocardiographic changes than are the other antipsychotic drugs, and in some patients it may be useful to do baseline electrocardiograms prior to treatment with these drugs.[6][7]

Anticholinergic Effects

All known antipsychotic drugs can produce anticholinergic, or atropine-like, effects.[5] These effects are generally manifested by blurred vision, dryness of the mouth, constipation, urinary retention, decreased perspiration, and increased heart rate. Usually these symptoms are simply unpleasant or annoying, but in certain patients they may be of more serious medical importance. Patients with narrow-angle glaucoma are particularly vulnerable to anticholinergic drug effects, which may produce an increase in intraocular pressure and worsen their condition.[5] Patients with coronary heart disease may also experience a worsening of symptoms (even angina) in the presence of drugs which induce tachycardia. On the other hand, antipsychotic drugs with higher anticholinergic potencies may also offer positive benefits. Recent studies indicate that those antipsychotic drugs with greater anticholinergic effects are less likely to induce extrapyramidal symptoms, and, indeed, this may explain the particularly low incidence of parkinsonian symptoms in patients receiving thioridazine.[8] Among the antipsychotic drugs, thioridazine is the most potent anticholinergic agent, and chlorpromazine is also rather strongly anticholinergic; trifluoperazine and fluphenazine are far less potent in their atropine-like effects; and haloperidol has the lowest anticholinergic potential.[5][8]

---

*Jerrold G. Bernstein 1973: unpublished observations.

It has been well known for over 100 years that atropine-like drugs can produce toxic symptoms, including an acute delirium or psychotic state.[5] Psychiatric patients are particularly vulnerable to toxic psychoses induced by therapeutic agents. At first it may seem paradoxical that a patient receiving a therapeutic dose of an antipsychotic drug suddenly appears to be more psychotic than at the outset of treatment. Again, however, an understanding of the pharmacology of the therapeutic agents makes this clinical situation readily understandable. If a patient's psychotic symptoms appear to worsen during the course of treatment with antipsychotic agents, one should first consider the possibility of an anticholinergic-induced delirium. Such a syndrome can be produced in certain patients by the more potent anticholinergic antipsychotic drugs, particularly thioridazine.

Antiparkinsonian drugs such as trihexyphenidyl (Artane) and benztropine (Cogentin), which are commonly used along with antipsychotic drugs, may also be responsible for drug-induced anticholinergic psychoses.[5] [9] Most antiparkinsonian drugs, except amantadine (Symmetrel) and L-dopa, exert their therapeutic effects primarily by means of their anticholinergic action.[5] Antiparkinsonian drugs exert strong peripheral anticholinergic effects that are likely to be manifested by the same symptoms of blurred vision, dry mouth, constipation, urinary retention, decreased perspiration, and tachycardia. These effects are, of course, additive with anticholinergic effects produced by the antipsychotic drugs. When a delirium or worsening of psychotic symptoms occurs in a patient being treated for psychosis, one should first discontinue any antiparkinsonian drugs. If the patient is receiving strongly anticholinergic antipsychotic medication, this, too, should be stopped and replaced by a less anticholinergic antipsychotic drug, such as trifluoperazine, fluphenazine, or haloperidol.

PERIPHERAL EFFECTS OF TRICYCLIC ANTIDEPRESSANTS AND THEIR MANAGEMENT

Anticholinergic Effects

The tricyclic antidepressant drugs are even more potent in their anticholinergic effects, both centrally and peripherally, than are the antipsychotic drugs.[5] [10] In certain susceptible individuals there is a very great likelihood of producing an exacerbation of psychotic symptoms by the administration of tricyclic antidepressant drugs. Even in occasional individuals who have no apparent underlying psychotic illness, acute toxic psychoses produced by pronounced cholinergic blockade may be observed with the tricyclic antidepressants. Among these drugs, amitriptyline (Elavil) has the greatest anticholinergic potential; imipramine has a somewhat lower anticholinergic potency; and doxepin is the least potent in this regard.

In view of the fact that so many of the drugs used in psychiatry do produce clinically significant anticholinergic effects, and that these drugs are often used in combination with each other, it is necessary to understand the principles of cholinergic blockade and additive drug interactions in this area of therapeutics.[1][11] Many of our patients may be taking other anticholinergic drugs, either in the course of medical treatment by other physicians, or illicitly, through channels of drug abuse. The best way to manage this problem is to take a careful drug history and ascertain that the patient is not receiving anticholinergic drugs from another physician or in the form of street drugs.

Next, the psychotropic drug regimen must be designed to minimize these unpleasant symptoms. Frequently phenothiazines will be used in conjunction with tricyclic antidepressants in order to achieve a better antidepressant response or to minimize anxiety. A patient receiving phenothiazines along with tricyclic antidepressants almost never requires antiparkinsonian medication, since the central atropine-like effect of therapeutic doses of the antidepressant usually counteracts parkinsonian symptoms.[1][5] A patient receiving tricyclic antidepressants alone, however, may complain of unpleasant physiologic symptoms related to anticholinergic effect. Such a patient may benefit from bethanecol (Urecholine) at an oral dosage of 10 to 25 mg two to four times per day.[12] Bethanecol is a potent and stable cholinergic stimulant which may, in some patients, overcome or reduce the severity of peripheral anticholinergic effects of antipsychotic and antidepressant drugs without decreasing their therapeutic efficacy. Patients receiving antipsychotic or antidepressant drugs who persistently complain of dry mouth may be helped by pilocarpine, 1% aqueous solution, at a dosage of 5 ml three or four times per day as a mouthwash and gargle.* This agent is a rather effective salivary stimulant.[13] If blurred vision produced by psychotropic drug treatment is severe enough to limit a patient's daily functioning, it may be overcome by one of two approaches. Eye drops containing 1% or 2% pilocarpine may be administered two or three times daily, or the patient may seek ophthalmologic consultation and be fitted for corrective lenses to be used during the course of psychotropic drug treatment.[14]

---

*Jerrold G. Bernstein 1974: unpublished observations.

Patients presenting with acute anticholinergic syndromes marked by delirium, confusion, and psychotic symptoms produced by therapeutic use of psychotropic drugs, accidental or intentional overdose of these drugs, or use of illicit "street" drugs may benefit greatly from physostigmine.[9] Physostigmine is a potent anticholinesterase drug which improves the physiology of cholinergic nerve transmission by temporarily inhibiting acetylcholine breakdown.[15] This compound is marketed in ampules containing 1 mg physostigmine per ml solution for intramuscular or intravenous injection. Physostigmine (Antilirium) can be injected intramuscularly in doses of 1 or 2 mg, or 1 mg of the drug may be diluted with saline solution to an injection volume of 10 ml, which may be given intravenously over two to five minutes. Generally, patients with drug-induced anticholinergic delirious states will improve significantly within 15 to 30 minutes after the injection, showing increased salivation and perspiration, a slowing of the heart rate, and a desire to urinate. If no effect is observed within 30 minutes after the initial 1-mg dose, a second 1-mg dose can be administered. If an effect is observed, it frequently will be relatively short-lived, because physostigmine is a short-acting reversible cholinesterase inhibitor. [9] [15] Thus, physostigmine can be helpful in making the initial diagnosis and in dictating therapy, which would typically include hospitalizing the patient briefly, withholding psychotropic drugs other than mild sedatives such as barbiturates or diazepam, administering physostigmine intramuscularly as required, and awaiting spontaneous clearing of symptoms, which could be expected to occur over 24 to 48 hours.

Cardiac Arrhythmias

Sinus tachycardia and changes in electrical impulse conduction within the heart may occur as a consequence of the anticholinergic actions of tricyclic antidepressants.[6] [10] Their anticholinergic actions are a part of the basic mechanism of action of these drugs, which are believed to exert their antidepressant effect by blocking nerve re-uptake of norepinephrine and thus increasing the availability of functional norepinephrine at nerve endings. This apparently occurs at various sites throughout the body, as well as in the brain, and patients receiving therapeutic doses of tricyclic antidepressants may develop cardiac arrythmias, particularly premature ventricular and premature atrial contractions, presumably as a result of increased norepinephrine in the myocardium.[10] These arrhythmias are most commonly seen in patients with underlying coronary heart disease or with preexisting disturbances of cardiac rhythm. Such patients should therefore be carefully screened and have baseline electrocardiograms before beginning therapy with these drugs. As these patients may be more likely to develop cardiac arrhythmias or experience a worsening of existing arrhythmias if the antidepressant drugs are given in large or in single daily doses at the outset of therapy, they should begin treatment with divided doses and gradually increase the total daily dosage until a therapeutic dosage is attained. Clinical experience suggests that doxepin (Sinequan) is less likely to induce or worsen cardiac arrhythmias than is amitriptyline (Elavil) or imipramine (Tofranil); thus doxepin might be the drug of choice in a susceptible individual. The initial dosage might be 25 mg two or three times daily, and dosage increases would optimally be followed by pulse measurements or electrocardiographic tracings. The lesser likelihood of cardiac arrhythmias associated with doxepin may be related to its weaker anticholinergic potency, since anticholinergic effects would act in an additive fashion with the tricyclics' increasing the availability of norepinephrine in the myocardium.[10]

Tricyclic antidepressants administered to animals in doses equivalent to human therapeutic doses have been documented as inducing myocardial depression and precipitating congestive heart failure.[10] There have been several reports in the literature of congestive heart failure occurring in patients receiving usual therapeutic doses of tricyclic antidepressants. Although this is a rather unusual finding with these drugs, it is not uncommon to see pedal edema in patients receiving tricyclic antidepressants, and this might represent evidence of mild, drug-induced congestive heart failure.[10]

Hypotension

Hypotensive responses to tricyclic antidepressants are quite common.[10] Usually the hypotension seen is in response to postural change and may therefore simply be postural hypotension in the presence of vasodilatation or impaired baroreceptor reflex function. On the other hand, since postural hypotension tends to occur more often in patients with underlying heart disease, it may stem from drug-related myocardial depression. Among the tricyclic antidepressants, doxepin is least likely to induce postural hypotension.

Despite all of these cautions, treatment with tricyclic antidepressants is not absolutely contraindicated in a patient with stable heart disease,[10] although it is generally advisable in such patients to employ the antidepressant least likely to induce cardiovascular effects (ie, doxepin) and to start with a relatively low dose and increase the dose gradually. Baseline electrocardiograms should be obtained in such patients, and electrocardiograms should be obtained serially during the course of dosage adjustments. In patients with significant cardiovascular disease, it may be advisable to begin treatment with tricyclic antidepressants while the patient is still in the hospital, where greater medical support is available.

Tricyclic Inhibition of Guanethidine

Tricyclic antidepressants may interfere with the drugs used to treat essential hypertension. This group of antidepressant drugs acts by blocking nerve re-uptake of norepinephrine, and one of the widely used antihypertensive medications, guanethidine (Ismelin), acts to lower blood pressure by first being taken up into adrenergic nerve endings by the same process that is involved in norepinephrine re-uptake. If this process is blocked by tricyclic antidepressants, guanethidine does not enter the nerve and is not able to exert its blood-pressure-lowering effect. Therefore, if a patient receiving guanethidine for blood pressure control is given a tricyclic antidepressant, his blood pressure will become uncontrolled and will continue to climb to hypertensive levels. Similarly, if a patient is receiving tricyclic antidepressants and is then given guanethidine for hypertension, the latter drug will be ineffective because of the failure of nerve tissue to take it up and utilize it.[10] The risks in combining guanethidine with tricyclic antidepressants are particularly great because if one is unaware of their peculiar interaction and proceeds to progressively increase the dose of guanethidine in an attempt to achieve a therapeutic effect, the patient may develop a severe hypotensive reaction should the tricyclic antidepressant be discontinued. It was formerly believed that doxepin did not interfere with the action of guanethidine, but more recent data confirms the finding that all tricyclic antidepressants have this effect. The antihypertensive action of clonidine (Catapres) is similarly inhibited by tricyclic antidepressants.[16]

Antihypertensive Agents and Tricyclic Treatment of Depression

Two widely used antihypertensive medications, methyldopa and reserpine, are capable of inducing depression, particularly in susceptible individuals with a prior history of affective illness.[10 17 18] Thus far, there is very little data to suggest that tricyclic antidepressants interfere with the hypotensive action of methyldopa, and therefore these two drugs can be used concurrently.[10] However, if a patient with both hypertension and depression does not show improvement of depressive symptoms despite the use of tricyclic antidepressants, one should seriously consider discontinuing the methyldopa and using another hypotensive agent, since the methyldopa may be exacerbating or inducing the depression.

Presently there are many effective antihypertensive medications available, and reserpine is not used as extensively as it once was. If a patient with clinical depression is receiving reserpine, the patient's internist should be consulted and his antihypertensive therapy changed, since the reserpine itself may be the major cause of the depression and it is easier to avoid this medication than to attempt to pharmacologically treat a drug-related depression.[17]

MAO INHIBITORS

Despite the fact that the tricyclic compounds are the most popular antidepressants in current use, there are some patients for whom treatment with monoamine oxidase (MAO) inhibitors offers certain advantages. The MAO inhibitors may be uniquely effective in some depressed patients who have failed to respond to the conventional tricyclic drugs.[19] [20] Furthermore, some recent data suggest that MAO inhibitors may have a particular advantage in the treatment of patients with phobic or obsessive-compulsive disorders.[21] Additionally, some patients are unable to tolerate the strong anticholinergic effects of the tricyclic drugs, and patients with prostatic enlargement may develop urinary retention on minimal, subtherapeutic doses of tricyclic compounds; therefore, we should not discard the MAO inhibitors and perhaps should use them more freely in selected patients.

This group of drugs has fallen out of favor primarily because of numerous reports in the literature of hypertensive crises, and even cerebrovascular accidents, occurring in patients treated with them. The hypertensive crises associated with MAO inhibitors occurred in patients known to have eaten certain tyramine-rich foods during therapy, or to have been concurrently using medications containing derivatives of phenylethylamine. Monoamine oxidase inhibitors exert their antidepressant action by inhibiting an enzyme which is important in the metabolism and breakdown of norepinephrine. This same enzyme is active in the metabolism of endogenous catecholamines as well as of phenylethylamine-type vasoconstrictor substances. Patients who are taking an MAO inhibiting drug and who eat tyramine-rich foods such as fermented cheese, red wine, or beer will show an increase in blood pressure which can be great enough to produce a cerebrovascular accident. Similarly, patients who receive MAO inhibitor drugs and also use medications such as nasal decongestant nose drops, patent cold remedies, or amphetamine-like weight-reducing products also risk hypertensive crises.

If there are clinical indications for treatment with an MAO inhibitor, and if the patient is reliable and is willing to follow certain dietary restrictions, these drugs can be used safely and effectively. It is of utmost importance, however, that the patient be carefully and completely informed as to the foods and medications that he must avoid.[19-22] The best practice is to provide the patient with a printed list of foods and medications that should be avoided and to periodically monitor the patient's blood pressure and reemphasize the need for abstinence from these foods and medications during the course of treatment with these very potent and effective drugs.

LITHIUM

Lithium carbonate is a mood-stabilizing drug and is among the most useful and important of the modern advances in psychopharmacology. Lithium is useful in the treatment of the manic phase of manic-depressive illness as well as in the prophylaxis of both mania and depression.[23] There is some data which suggest that lithium is also useful adjunctively in the treatment of depression and that it may be of considerable value in the treatment of less clear-cut disorders of mood and impulse control, including emotionally unstable character disorders.[24] [25]

Lithium is unique in that it is a simple ion rather than a complex molecule like all other psychoactive drugs. It is also unique in that it produces few, if any, subjective effects in the average patient. Patients receiving this drug do not feel "medicated," mentally dulled, sedated, or stimulated. Yet its effects are profound, and if not adequately respected and carefully used, it can produce toxic side effects.[26] The most common side effects of lithium include heartburn and mild nausea. Fortunately, these effects are also the easiest to treat, since they generally disappear if the patient takes lithium along with meals or a snack. Many patients will have a fine resting tremor of the hand when they first begin treatment with lithium. This generally disappears within two or three weeks, but in some cases it may persist throughout the treatment, even when the dosage is changed to produce lower blood levels. Antiparkinsonian drugs have no effect on this tremor because it is not a parkinsonian tremor. Propranolol (Inderal), a beta-adrenergic blocking agent, is highly effective in eliminating lithium-induced finger tremors in virtually all patients.

Propranolol is a potent drug which must be used under careful medical supervision because of its ability to slow the heart, lower blood pressure, and impair pulmonary function in susceptible individuals. Generally, doses of 10 to 20 mg of propranolol three to four times daily will rapidly extinguish lithium-induced tremors.[27]

A baseline electrocardiogram should be done prior to starting treatment with lithium as it can induce cardiac arrhythmias or worsen preexisting arrhythmias in some people. Furthermore, lithium may produce electrocardiographic changes which resemble those of hypokalemia, including changes in the T wave and ST segment.[26] The baseline electrocardiogram will not only help to rule out prior abnormalities, but it will also serve as a point of comparison should electrocardiographic abnormalities be noted during treatment with lithium.

Lithium is filtered, reabsorbed, and excreted by the kidney similarly to sodium.[23] It is therefore important to obtain serum creatinine and/or blood urea nitrogen (BUN) measurements prior to instituting lithium treatment because impaired renal function may lead to unanticipated high blood levels of lithium and consequent lithium toxicity. Lithium frequently produces an increase in urinary output and an associated increase in thirst. These symptoms are generally fairly mild, and though at times inconvenient, they have no serious consequences and do not necessitate discontinuance of lithium therapy. In rare patients, a syndrome resembling nephrogenic diabetes insipidus, with intense thirst and the production of large volumes of very dilute urine, develops. This syndrome is generally reversible in a relatively short time after discontinuance of lithium therapy.[23] [26] However, some patients who develop this syndrome have had such a strikingly beneficial response to lithium that we may wish to continue therapy despite the diabetes insipidus—like syndrome. Such continued treatment with lithium is not contraindicated. In some cases, the lithium-induced diabetes insipidus—like syndrome responds favorably to thiazide diuretics, which effect a paradoxical antidiuretic response. This syndrome is not reversed, however, by vasopressin.

Rarely, in patients receiving lithium over a prolonged period, mild hypothyroidism develops. In other patients, benign, diffuse enlargement of the thyroid gland develops, though the patient remains euthyroid. There is no particular danger to the patient who develops lithium-induced thyroid changes, although in some cases the patient may benefit clinically if given thyroid hormone in conjunction with continued lithium therapy.[23] [26]

Many patients receiving lithium over a prolonged period experience mild to moderate weight gain, frequently in association with peripheral edema. Although one must be cautious in the concurrent use of lithium and diuretics—since diuretics, as well as salt-restricted diets, can lead to increased serum lithium levels—clinical studies have documented that spironolactone (Aldactone) may be used safely in conjuction with lithium as a means of reducing lithium-induced peripheral edema.[28]

REFERENCES

1. Byck, R.: Drugs and the treatment of psychiatric disorders. In Goodman, L.S. and Gilman, A. (eds.): *The Pharmacological Basis of Therapeutics.* 5th ed. New York: MacMillan Publishing Co., 1975.

2. Snyder, S.H.: The dopamine hypothesis of schizophrenia: focus on the dopamine receptor. *Am. J. Psychiatry* 133:197-202, 1976.

3. Snyder, S.H., Banerjee, S.P., Yamamura, H.I. et al: Drugs, neurotransmitters, and schizophrenia. *Science* 184:1234-1253, 1974.

4. Seeman, P. and Lee, T.: Antipsychotic drugs: direct correlation between clinical potency and presynaptic actions on dopamine neurons. *Science* 188:1217-1219, 1975.

5. Shader, R.I. and DiMascio, A.: *Psychotropic Drug Side Effects.* Baltimore: The Williams & Wilkins Co., 1970.

6. Fowler, N.O., McCall, D., Chou, T.C., et al: Electrocardiographic changes and cardiac arrhythmias in patients receiving psychotropic drugs. *Am. J. Cardiol.* 37:223-230, 1976.

7. Ban, T.A. and St. Jean, A.: The effects of phenothiazines on the electrocardiogram. *Can. Med. Assoc. J.* 91:537-540, 1964.

8. Snyder, S., Greenberg, D., and Yamamura, H.I.: Antischizophrenic drugs and brain cholinergic receptors. *Arch. Gen. Psychiatry* 31:58-61, 1974.

9. Granacher, R.P. and Baldessarini, R.J.: Physostigmine. *Arch. Gen. Psychiatry* 32:375-380, 1975.

10. Jefferson, J.W: A review of the cardiovascular effects and toxicity of tricyclic antidepressants. *Psychosom. Med.* 37:160-179, 1975.

11. Innes, I.R. and Nickerson, M.: Atropine, scopolamine, and related antimuscarinic drugs. In Goodman, L.S. and Gilman, A. (eds.): *The Pharmacological Basis of Therapeutics.* 5th ed. New York: MacMillan Publishing Co., 1975, pp. 514-532.

12. Everett, H.C.: The use of bethanechol chloride with tricyclic antidepressants. *Am. J. Psychiatry* 132:1202-1204, 1975.

13. Koelle, G.B.: Parasympathomimetic agents. In Goodman, L.S. and Gilman, A. (eds.): *The Pharmacological Basis of Therapeutics.* 5th ed. New York: MacMillan Publishing Co., 1975, pp. 467-476.

14. Bassuk, E.L. and Schoonover, S.C.: *The Practitioner's Guide to Psychoactive Drugs.* New York: Plenum Press, 1977, p. 95.

15. Koelle, G.B.: Anticholinesterase agents. In Goodman, L.S. and Gilman, A. (eds.): *The Pharmacological Basis of Therapeutics.* 5th ed. New York: MacMillan Publishing Co., 1975, pp. 445-466.

16. Briant, R.H., Reid, J.L., and Dolery, C.T.: Interaction between clonidine and desipramine in man. *Br. Med. J.* 1:522-523, 1973.

17. Quetsch, R.M., Achor, R.W.P., Litin, E.M. et al: Depressive reaction in hypertensive patients: a comparison of those treated with rauwolfia and those receiving no specific antihypertensive treatment. *Circulation* 19:366-375, 1959.

18. McKinney, W.P., Jr. and Kane, F.J., Jr.: Depression with the use of alpha-methyldopa. *Am. J. Psychiatry* 124: 80-81, 1967.

19. Lurie, M.L. and Salzer, H.M.: Tranylcypromine (Parnate) in the ambulatory treatment of depressed patients. *Am. J. Psychiatry* 118:152-155, 1961.

20. Today's drugs: Monoamine oxidase inhibitors, editorial. *Br. Med. J.* 1:35-37, 1968.

21. Robinson, D.S., Nies, A., Lamborn, K.R. et al: Controlled clinical trial of the MAO inhibitor phenelzine in the treatment of depressive-anxiety states. *Arch. Gen. Psychiatry* 29:407-416, 1973.

22. Spiker, D.G. and Pugh, D.D.: Combining tricyclic and monoamine oxidase inhibitor antidepressants. *Arch. Gen. Psychiatry* 33:828-830, 1976.

23. Baldessarini, R.J. and Lipinski, J.F.: Lithium salts: 1970-1975. *Ann. Intern. Med.* 83:527-533, 1975.

24. Noyes, R., Jr., Dempsey, G.M., Blum, A. et al: Lithium treatment of depression. *Comp. Psychiatry* 15:187-193, 1974.

25. Rifkin, A., Quitkin, F., Carrillo, C. et al: Lithium carbonate in emotionally unstable character disorder. *Arch. Gen. Psychiatry* 27:519-523, 1972.

26. Shopsin, B. and Gershon, S.: Pharmacology-toxicology of the lithium ion. In Gershon, S., and Shopsin, B. (eds.): *Lithium: Its Role in Psychiatric Research and Treatment.* New York: Plenum Press, 1973, pp. 107-146.

27. Kirk, L. Baastrup, P.C. and Schou, M.: Propranolol treatment of lithium-induced tremor. *Lancet* II:1086, 1973.

28. Demers, R. and Heninger, G.: Pretibial edema and sodium retention during lithium carbonate treatment. *JAMA.* 214:1845-1848, 1970.

11 Drug Abuse Problems and Their Management

John C. Kuehnle, M.D.

The clinical problems of drug abuse are those of intoxication and withdrawal. Knowledge of the effects of intoxication and withdrawal of a drug enables an understanding of what is happening, at least biologically, with an individual who has abused the drug.[1]

NARCOTICS

A wide variety of natural and synthetic narcotics are abused by members of the drug culture. Heroin and methadone are of particular importance in this regard, and a comparison of their characteristics is essential to understanding the clinical problem of narcotic addiction. Heroin is a shorter-acting drug than methadone and it shows an earlier onset of withdrawal symptoms. While heroin withdrawal begins 12 to 14 hours after administration (this time may vary; the more potent the heroin, the more delayed the onset of withdrawal) and peaks in 36 to 72 hours, methadone withdrawal begins much later and lasts much longer. It may take as long as 6 days for the methadone withdrawal reaction to peak, and the entire withdrawal period can last 10 to 14 days.[1]

In evaluating a drug addict, one must know the difference between signs and symptoms. In general, substances with a longer duration of action will have fewer symptoms, but these will last longer. The short-acting drugs produce a more severe, but shorter-lasting, withdrawal.

Signs and Symptoms of Withdrawal

Among the early signs of withdrawal are lacrimation, rhinorrhea, yawning, increased perspiration, restlessness, pupillary dilation, and piloerection. Dilated pupils and rhinorrhea are the two most common signs,[1] and the patient who claims to be in narcotic withdrawal should exhibit them (if he does not, there is a good chance he is not in withdrawal). Piloerection will be evident at the peak of withdrawal. Later, the patient may vomit. Vomiting, diarrhea, tachycardia, increased blood pressure, tremor, muscle spasms, and kicking movements of the legs are signs of severe withdrawal.[1]

The symptoms are quite variable and are seen long before the signs of withdrawal. They include increased irritability, insomnia, decreased appetite, feelings of restlessness, weakness, depression, abdominal pain, and leg cramps.[1] Cramping in the legs has always been present in heroin withdrawal, yet for some reason many methadone users claim that it is due to cancer of the bone. There is no evidence, however, to indicate that methadone does anything to bone tissue.[1]

When treating a methadone or heroin addict in an emergency situation, one should keep a few things in mind. In general, one never sees the addict while he is using his drug. Once, however, he begins withdrawal—or thinks he is beginning withdrawal—he will proceed to any place where he thinks he can acquire drugs. An important thing to remember when the addict comes into the hospital or clinic is that narcotic withdrawal is not a life-threatening situation.[1] If a person is in good health and does not have some severe, intercurrent illness, he will not die during withdrawal. Although he may complain a lot and be in great distress, the symptoms are probably equivalent to a bad case of the flu, and if for some reason you cannot get him methadone, he will survive.

To distinguish between an addict genuinely in withdrawal and a "copping junkie," one must look for objective signs, not just symptoms. Symptoms occur before withdrawal begins, and there is no way to validate them without looking closely for signs of withdrawal as the patient is examined. Some addicts will go to incredible lengths. A classic example occurred at Boston City Hospital several years ago. In this case a drug addict managed to get a five-day supply of methadone because he was flying to Rome to visit his dying mother. He had the methadone prescription filled, sold the drug, and then bought heroin, which he used. He then came back to the clinic five days later and explained very calmly what he had done. He had, in fact, bought airline tickets so that the doctor would believe that he was going to Rome, and after getting his methadone, he simply returned the tickets, got the money back, and also sold all the methadone.*

This is not an unusual situation; addicts are extremely resourceful individuals. In general, it is best to refer these patients to a specialized clinic. In an emergency situation, or where an immediate referral cannot be made, the most humane approach may be to provide treatment with methadone while the patient awaits transfer to a specialized facility.

Treatment of Withdrawal

In treating addicted patients, one should not prescribe any drug that can be abused. Specifically, avoid prescribing stimulants and sedative-hypnotic type drugs. If methadone must be given, it should be either in liquid form, or crushed and made to be swallowed with liquid. If it is in any other oral form, an addict will cheek it or put it under his tongue and save it, and he will later sell it so he can purchase heroin. This precaution may seem a little dramatic, but it can reduce the chances that more addicts will come back to attempt to cop drugs.

Addicts report that times have changed in the drug business. They say that, years ago, if an addict went to a general practitioner and complained about severe flank pains radiating down into his testicle, the physician would send him to the bathroom to give a urine specimen and the drug addict would simply prick his finger and squeeze a little blood into the urine. When the physician found the blood, he would make a diagnosis of renal colic and write a prescription for meperidine. Addicts no longer use this approach because they claim physicians are now more enlightened, and when a patient says that he is a junkie and needs prescriptions, the physicians often comply. Although they cannot easily get methadone prescriptions, sometimes the other prescriptions can be traded for narcotics on the street.

Methadone is the treatment of choice for narcotic withdrawal, and as is the strategy in treating any case of drug withdrawal, one titrates

---

*John Kuehnle 1972: personal observation.

the dose to achieve a balance between withdrawal and intoxication.[2] It is best to verify a patient's dosage if he has been in a methadone maintenance program. If the dosage cannot be verified, no more than 20 mg of methadone should be given initially.[1][2] The patient should then be observed for about two hours. If in that time the pupils constrict to pinpoint size and the individual appears very pleasant, rather than irritable, he has not been on methadone at all, and the 20-mg dose has given him a brief "high." If, however, the pupils remain dilated and the patient continues to be restless and to exhibit rhinorrhea and slight tachycardia, he may be administered another 20 mg. Titration of dosage should continue until the pupils and pulse rate are normalized.

The dose necessary to relieve the objective signs of withdrawal becomes the initial daily dosage for detoxification; this generally will not exceed 40 mg. (The early methadone maintenance programs often provided excessive doses and, also, take-home methadone. Empirical observations and controlled clinical trials demonstrated that individuals on dosages of up to 90 mg per day could get by on 40 mg per day if necessary. Often these patients would take the extra 50 mg and sell it so that they could buy heroin, which they preferred.) In an inpatient setting, detoxification can be effected by 5-mg decrements in dosage daily over a period of 7 to 10 days.[1][2] Adjunctive medication during or following detoxification should generally be avoided. Flurazepam or diphenhydramine, however, may be temporarily useful as an aid in providing sleep, although the former should be used cautiously as it has a potential for abuse. Haloperidol, in doses of 2 to 10 mg one to four times per day, is safe, and it may help reduce agitation that may occur during drug withdrawal. Flurazepam, diazepam, and other drugs with abuse potential should not be prescribed for the patient after his release from the hospital, as he may use them himself or sell them in order to obtain other drugs.

Overdosage

An addicted patient who is in a coma and has pinpoint pupils and depressed respiration has probably taken an overdose.[1][2] Naloxone reverses this very quickly, but it is important to remember that naloxone has a duration of action of about 3 to 4 hours, and the duration of action of methadone is about 24 hours. Therefore, if the patient has taken an overdose of methadone, he may become perfectly clear, alert, and responsive after intravenous administration of naloxone, and be in a coma again 5 hours later. Since the duration of action of heroin is short, recurrence of coma following naloxone reversal of heroin overdose presents few long-range problems. If the coma is due to methadone overdose, however, the patient requires careful observation and frequent administration of naloxone over a period of 12 to 24 hours or longer.[1][2]

The main source of other medical complications associated with heroin use is contaminated needles. When treating addicted patients, one should always consider the possible presence of hepatitis, septicemia, tetanus, brain abscess, subacute bacterial endocarditis, malaria, and other illnesses deriving from this source. Patients generally should be given a tetanus booster as a precaution.

ANTIANXIETY AGENTS

The antianxiety agents are the most widely used of the psychotropic drugs. The benzodiazepines diazepam (Valium) and chlordiazepoxide (Librium) are the medications prescribed most often, but sales of barbiturates and other sedatives are also extensive. These drugs are all pharmacologically similar and are best classified as sedative-hypnotic drugs. Their pharmacologic properties vary somewhat, but they are more similar than dissimilar, and cross tolerance is seen within the group.[1] High enough doses of these drugs will produce intoxication, and patients may develop withdrawal symptoms upon sudden discontinuation of a drug after long-term treatment.[3][4]

The benzodiazepines, the most widely used antianxiety drugs, have a temporary, anxiety-relieving effect at doses that do not produce profound sedation.[4] Anxiety-relieving doses of the barbiturates generally produce greater sedation, although some claim that the sedative effects of phenobarbital are less pronounced than those of the other barbiturates. Emergency room treatment of an acute anxiety reaction should consist of limited amounts of diazepam or chlordiazepoxide. These are best prescribed on an as-needed basis, because regular ingestion increases the blood levels of the drugs and results in drug tolerance and a loss of therapeutic effect. Also, patients chronically kept on these drugs tend to develop greater anxiety following dosage reduction or discontinuation.[3][5]

Physicians tend to prescribe diazepam and chlordiazepoxide rather liberally for presumed hypochondriacs. These patients often possess a variety of somatic complaints that have no discernible biologic bases, and the antianxiety drug treatment they receive is often excessive. Many of these individuals may have affective illness, and a very careful history should be taken to clarify this question. Any family history of alcoholism, depression, or suicide strengthens this possibility. Abnormalities in the sleep pattern also suggest affective illness. (If a patient is having difficulty falling asleep, one should verify whether or not he is taking any medication for this. A patient may report having no difficulties with sleep, but he may also be taking sedatives every night that have been prescribed by another doctor.) The presence of a sleep disorder and a loss of interest and energy, together with the patient's somatic symptoms, would suggest a diagnosis of depression. Such a patient deserves a trial with an anti-depressant, which can be discontinued if ineffective and which may prove much more beneficial than the chronic use of either diazepam or chlordiazepoxide.

The benzodiazepines, as do all drugs, carry both advantages and disadvantages.[4] A primary advantage of the benzodiazepines is their high margin of safety: they have very long half-lives, and this is not often appreciated. The half-life of chlordiazepoxide, for example, is about 24 hours.[4] Diazepam actually has two half-lives: the first begins when the drug is first ingested; the second, as it is stored in fat tissue, and it lasts until all of the stored drug has been metabolized. The first half-life can be very short—7 to 10 hours—while the second one lasts much longer—up to 50 hours.[4] There has been an apparent reduction in the number of successful suicides by drug overdose because of these drugs' high margin of safety. Death from overdose is much less likely with the benzodiazepines than with the barbiturates.[1][4] Unfortunately, there is a tendency on the part of some physicians to administer these drugs rather casually. Studies in hospitals have shown that the benzo-diazepines are more often prescribed by surgeons, internists, and general practitioners than by psychiatrists.[6]

Among the other critical things to know about these drugs is that they are very poorly absorbed when given by intramuscular injection (it can take up to several days for intramuscular doses of diazepam or chlordiazepoxide to be absorbed).[7] Therefore, the benzodiazepines should generally be given by mouth. If a rapid effect is desired, 5 mg of diazepam, or 10 to 15 mg of chlordiazepoxide, can be given intra-venously. When administering either of these intravenously, one should be prepared to breathe the patient; respiratory depression is rare, but it can occur.[1] It is also not generally appreciated that antacids greatly inhibit the absorption of benzodiazepines through the gastrointestinal tract.[4] This lack of knowledge constitutes a major stumbling block to effective treatment, as diazepam and chlordiaze-poxide are often given with over-the-counter antacid mixtures.

Intoxication and Withdrawal

The number-one drug of abuse in methadone clinics today is not heroin or alcohol, but diazepam. About one third of all patients in methadone clinics are taking diazepam—not always at high doses, but almost always illegally. Normal doses of benzodiazepines produce relaxation; larger doses produce euphoria and gregariousness. As the dose increases, dysphoria and nystagmus tend to develop. Nystagmus is a key sign of intoxication with benzodiazepines, barbiturates, or any of the sedative-hypnotics.[1] At larger doses, ataxia and unsteady gait develop. One can detect cases of overdoses of these drugs by looking for lateral gaze nystagmus and ataxia. At the far end of the dosage spectrum, stupor and coma are produced.

Withdrawal from the central nervous system depressants parallels narcotic withdrawal in that the shorter-acting drugs show a more acute but shorter-lasting withdrawal.[1] The longer-acting, more slowly excreted drugs will give milder withdrawal symptoms over a longer period of time. It also takes longer to develop a withdrawal syndrome with the long-acting drugs. The short-acting barbiturates include secobarbital and pentobarbital; alcohol could also be considered one of the short-acting sedative drugs. The onset of withdrawal would be within 4 to 6 hours with these short-acting drugs, and within 1 to 3 days with diazepam, chlordiazepoxide, or phenobarbital. The peak of withdrawal occurs within 1 to 7 days with the short-acting drugs and within 5 to 7 days with the longer-acting drugs. Withdrawal may continue for 15 days (fewer with the short-acting drugs, and from 5 to 20 days with the long-acting agents).

The most serious aspect of the withdrawal process of these drugs is the occurrence of seizures. Severely intoxicated patients must be hospitalized to be withdrawn. Smith and Wesson have previously employed outpatient detoxification for sedative-dependent patients.[8] They have since said they'd much rather hospitalize patients than try to treat them as outpatients. Seizures are much more likely to occur in withdrawal from the short-acting sedatives than from the long-acting ones. There are minor and major signs and symptoms.[9] The minor ones include anxiety, postural faintness, diaphoresis, coarse rhythmic intention tremor, insomnia, anorexia, vomiting, and muscular twitches. These symptoms are similar to those of narcotic withdrawal to some extent. The major signs are fever, delirium, and seizures. Hyperactive deep tendon reflexes are an early indication that the patient's condition will become serious;[9] the person will probably not convulse if he has normal deep tendon reflexes in the arms. Patellar reflexes are not a reliable index because they may be absent with thiamine deficiency. Patellar reflexes can appear relatively normal and the patient may still get into trouble.

Grand mal seizures are those most typically reported in association with sedative-hypnotic withdrawal, but peculiar minor motor seizures which are not part of the more classical grand mal seizure pattern may also occur.[9] Bernstein has observed a wide variety of tonic, clonic, and other, less impressive abnormal motor movements following withdrawal of these drugs.* Often these odd movements may be mistaken for a "faked" seizure, even by competent neurologists. Bizarre behavioral symptoms, including delirium and psychotic symptomatology, may appear as delayed indications of sedative withdrawal as late as 3 to 8 days after drug discontinuation. Clinical pictures resembling delirium tremens and Korsakoff's syndrome may occur. High fevers of up to 106°F may be a late-appearing and often irreversibly damaging manifestation of barbiturate or sedative withdrawal.[9]

How much medication has to be taken and for how long in order to evoke withdrawal symptoms upon discontinuation of the drug? As little as 15 mg of diazepam daily taken over a four-month period has been reported to have produced signs of minor withdrawal.[5] (These signs and symptoms resemble those of anxiety—insomnia, restlessness, tremor, and postural faintness—so when they appear, there is a tendency to give *more* of the drug.) Research studies with secobarbital show that 600 to 800 mg daily over a period of 35 to 57 days can produce major withdrawal signs and symptoms.[9] Therefore, all sedative-hypnotics should be dispensed very carefully—in minimal dosage, for a limited time.

Treatment of Withdrawal

In treating withdrawal, a test dose of the drug is administered to determine tolerance. If nystagmus, ataxia, or sedation occurs, the dose is excessive; hyperreflexia and strong deep tendon reflexes indicate that the test dose is too low. The tolerance test employs a short-acting barbiturate such as pentobarbital or secobarbital in an oral dose of 100 or 200 mg.[9] If the patient cannot take the medication orally, it is given intramuscularly. The 100-mg dose is administered every hour until the patient is mildly intoxicated: mild nystagmus develops; speech may become slightly slurred; the patient feels more relaxed.[9] If the patient shows signs of intoxication (sedation and nystagmus) after only one 100-mg dose of oral pentobarbital, he is not physically dependent and does not need further titration—he certainly does not need barbiturate withdrawal treatment.[9] On the other hand, if the patient is addicted and does need a significant dose of barbiturate to demonstrate drug effect, gradual withdrawal will be required. The initial daily dosage of pentobarbital should be four times the dose needed to produce nystagmus during the tolerance test.[9]

---

*Jerrold Bernstein 1972: unpublished observations.

The patient should be monitored for a day or two until his condition has stabilized. Then the gradual withdrawal of the drug can begin. The daily dosage should not be reduced by more than 10% per day, as withdrawal at a rate faster than this risks the development of withdrawal symptoms.[9] Generally, pentobarbital would be reduced by 100 mg a day. If signs of withdrawal appear, increase the dosage by about 100 mg, hold it at this level for a day or two, and then start reducing it by 50-mg daily decrements.

An alternative method uses phenobarbital to replace the other drugs: 30 mg of phenobarbital is equal to 100 mg of secobarbital or pentobarbital, 10 mg of diazepam, 25 mg of chlordiazepoxide, or 400 mg of meprobamate.[8] If phenobarbital is substituted for pentobarbital, it can be administered in three or four divided doses each day and the total daily dosage can be reduced by 30 mg daily. Phenobarbital is much longer acting than pentobarbital, and it also has a direct anticonvulsant effect.[1][8]

When a patient has abused both narcotics and central nervous system depressants, it is best to withdraw the depressant first, as withdrawal from depressants is more dangerous and carries more risk than withdrawal from narcotics. Also, many of these individuals leave the hospital against medical advice, and if they leave under these conditions, they are better off having first completed barbiturate detoxification. Their methadone withdrawal can be carried out on an outpatient basis.

MARIJUANA

The narcotics and the antianxiety agents produce definable objective signs and symptoms of intoxication and withdrawal; these reactions are not so clear-cut with marijuana. Marijuana intoxication tends to be difficult to define if one has not experienced it, and even many who have experienced it have a difficult time describing it. Withdrawal symptoms with marijuana are virtually unheard of. Although Jones claims that marijuana can produce a withdrawal syndrome identical to that of the barbiturates, other researchers have not found this.[10][11]

Reactions to smoking marijuana fall into two broad groups: acute and chronic. There is not much controversy over acute reactions, which are easy to document: an individual exhibits no pathology before he smokes; he smokes, and some pathology appears; he stops smoking, and the pathology retreats. This is a clear-cut sequence that everyone can agree on. The implications for society of the short-term, or acute, reactions are not very profound. Weil has described depressive reactions to smoking marijuana; he observes that most of these occur in people with obsessive-compulsive tendencies.[12]

These individuals have a hard time enjoying smoking, and smoking makes them somewhat depressed. Panic reactions are the most common of the acute reactions, and they generally occur in novice smokers.[13][14] When these subjects experience changes in their perceptions and in their sense of time, they develop tachycardia and a feeling of anxiety. This escalates, and they often think they are losing their minds. These reactions should be treated not with medication but simply with reassurance. The setting and the expectations and personality of the individual are considered major determinants for the possible development of a panic reaction to marijuana (eg, a panic reaction would be likely should there be a police raid). Toxic psychosis, on the other hand, is thought to result principally from the action of the drug, and is therefore a reaction almost any individual could experience.[14] It is not a reaction likely to occur in smoking marijuana, however, because the process of intoxication is slow enough that one can titrate his intake of the drug much better than one can, for example, with oral hashish or hashish oil. According to the current literature, no one has ever died of an overdose of marijuana that has been smoked, but serious reactions have occurred with absorption of large oral doses of hashish oil.[15]

Among the chronic reactions, flashbacks have been reported, but the validity of these is still somewhat controversial.[14][16] One of the greater controversies revolves around whether long-term use of marijuana produces either a schizophrenia-like psychosis or an amotivational syndrome. McLaughlin and West coined the term "amotivational syndrome," and other investigators pointed out the danger of marijuana use producing psychosis or ruining careers.[13][16][17] They generally draw from select samples, and in all probability, the cases they so diagnose are variations of manic-depressive illness or schizophrenia, the onset of which coincides with a rather long-term use of marijuana. Psychotic illnesses can emerge from a variety of circumstances, but if marijuana is being used, and if one has a high index of suspicion for marijuana, one tends to blame marijuana. Extensive studies in Jamaica, Costa Rica, and Greece, however, in which very high doses of marijuana have been consumed for prolonged periods, failed to demonstrate that a psychotic condition results from its chronic use.[18]

Investigating the possibility of cerebral damage from marijuana use, Campbell et al did pneumoencephalographic studies of heavy cannabis users and found evidence of brain atrophy.[19] Attempts to replicate that study using the more sensitive technique of computerized axial tomography (known as CAT-scan), however, have not demonstrated any cerebral atrophic changes.[20][21]

144

In general, marijuana as presently consumed in the United States appears to be a mild intoxicant with potentially adverse acute effects and questionable long-term effects. Of course, chronic intoxication or frequent acute intoxication with any drug would indicate that an individual may have a number of problems which may be equally significant whether they preceded his drug abuse or proceed from it.

REFERENCES

1. Jaffe, J.H.: Drug addiction and drug abuse. In Goodman, L.S. and Gilman, A.: (eds.): *The Pharmacological Basis of Therapeutics.* 5th ed. New York: MacMillan Publishing Co., 1975, pp. 284-324.

2. Freedman, A.M.: Opiate dependence. In Freedman, A.M., Kaplan, H.I., and Sadock, B.J. (eds.): *Comprehensive Textbook of Psychiatry.* 2d ed. Baltimore: The Williams & Wilkins Co., 1975, pp. 1298-1317.

3. Covi, L. et al: Length of treatment with anxiolytic sedatives and response to their sudden withdrawal. *Acta Psychiatr. Scand.* 49:51-64, 1973.

4. Greenblatt, D.J. and Shader, R.I.: Benzodiazepines. *N. Engl. J. Med.* 291:19, 1011-1015, 1974.

5. Haskell, D.: Withdrawal of diazepam. *JAMA.* 233:135, 1975.

6. Wheatley, D.: *Psychopharmacology in Family Practice.* London: William Heinemann Medical Books Ltd., 1973.

7. Greenblatt, D.J. et al: Slow absorption of intramuscular chlordiazepoxide. *N. Engl. J. Med.* 291:21, 1116-1118, 1974.

8. Smith, D.E. and Wesson, D.R.: A new method for treatment of barbiturate dependence. *JAMA.* 213:294-295, 1970.

9. Wikler, A.: Diagnosis and treatment of drug dependence of the barbiturate type. *Am. J. Psychiatry* 125:6, 758-764, 1968.

10. Jones, R.T., Benowitz, N., and Bachman, J.: Clinical studies of cannabis tolerance and dependence. *Ann. N.Y. Acad. Sci.* 282:221-239, 1976.

11. Babor, T.F., Mendelson, J.H., Greenberg, I. et al: Marijuana consumption and the development of tolerance to physiological and subjective effects. *Arch. Gen. Psychiatry* 32:1548-1552, 1975.

12. Weil, A.T.: Adverse reactions to marijuana: classification and suggested treatment. *N. Engl. J. Med.* 282:997-1000, 1970.

13. McLaughlin, W.H. and West, L.J.: The marijuana problem: an overview. *Am. J. Psychiatry* 125:126-134, 1968.

14. Beaubrun, M.H. and Knight, F.: Psychiatric assessment of thirty chronic users of cannabis and thirty matched controls. *Am. J. Psychiatry* 130:309-311, 1973.

15. Lopez, H.H., Jr., Goldman, S.M., Liberman, I.I. et al: Cannabis—accidental peroral intoxication. *JAMA.* 227:1041-1042, 1974.

16. Halikas, J.A., Goodwin, D.W., and Guze, S.B.: Marihuana use and psychiatric illness. *Arch. Gen. Psychiatry* 27:162-165, 1972.

17. Kupfer, D.H., Detre, T., Koral, J. et al: A comment on the amotivational syndrome in marijuana smokers. *Am. J. Psychiatry* 130:1319-1322, 1973.

18. Chopra, G.S. and Smith, J.W.: Psychotic reactions following cannabis use in East Indians. *Arch. Gen. Psychiatry* 30:24-27, 1974.

19. Campbell, A.N.G., Evans, M., Thomson, J.L.G. et al: Cerebral atrophy in young cannabis smokers. *Lancet* II:1219-1224, 1971.

20. Kuehnle, J.C., Mendelson, J.H., Davis, K.R. et al: Computed tomographic examination of heavy marijuana smokers. *JAMA.* 237:1231-1232, 1977.

21. Co, B.T., Goodwin, D.W., Gado, M. et al: Absence of cerebral atrophy in chronic cannabis users. *JAMA.* 237:1229-1230, 1977.

12 The Right to Know: A Patient's Guide to Psychotropic Medications

Jerrold G. Bernstein, M.D.

INTRODUCTION

Of all the fields of medical practice, psychiatry is perhaps the most dependent upon patient cooperation and the participation of the individual in his or her own treatment. As is well recognized, psychotherapy is a process which involves "work" by the patient as well as by the therapist. Furthermore, drug treatment in psychiatry, as in other fields of medicine, hinges on the patient's following instructions and taking his or her medications according to prescription. There has been extensive discussion in the medical literature of the problem of noncompliance with recommended therapeutic regimens. No matter how effective a medication may be, the benefit is ultimately dependent upon the medication being consumed properly by the patient, and the likelihood of a patient following a recommended regimen of drug treatment is often directly related to that patient's understanding of his or her treatment. Clinical experience and research studies support the notion that patients who understand their treatment are more apt to take their medication properly and thereby achieve greater therapeutic benefit.[1]

145

The question of how much information patients need remains under debate, yet it seems reasonable that a physician provide his patients with enough information to allow them to understand as well as possible the nature of their illness. When one treats a patient with medication, it is important to share with that patient what one expects to accomplish by giving the medication. Furthermore, the patient should know the nature of side effects or complications that may be associated with the recommended treatment. It is important to present this information in terms understandable to the patient and to allow the patient an opportunity to discuss the information and to clarify it according to his or her own needs. Patients who are relatively sophisticated may require in-depth information and may ask for references to scientific articles; some may even read such technical articles on their own and ask to discuss them. Other patients may ask for written material specifically prepared for laymen to help them understand their treatment. There are also those patients who will clearly have questions in mind but will be reticent to verbalize them because they do not want to put their physician "on the spot." This chapter is intended as a guide to meeting the needs of these patients by presenting some of the current concepts of psychiatric treatment in a form understandable to laymen.

OVERVIEW

Many patients ask, "If I am feeling depressed or am having difficulties in my life, why should I take medicine?" Many things may be said in answer to such a question. First of all, life's problems are not always solved by medication, and indeed, many problems for which patients consult mental health professionals do not require treatment with medication. However, certain psychiatric conditions are believed to be related to chemical or biologic abnormalities in brain function: there is considerable evidence that abnormal brain chemistry is a significant factor in depression, mania, and psychotic disorders such as schizophrenia.[2] One of the most significant advances in psychiatry during the last 25 years has been the development of a wide range of compounds which are highly effective and beneficial in the treatment of many of these emotional and psychiatric disorders. These compounds fall into four basic classes: (1) antianxiety agents; (2) antipsychotics; (3) antidepressants; and (4) mood-stabilizing drugs. The majority of these medications act chemically or physiologically to change brain function, and they have been demonstrated to counteract many of the symptoms and feelings associated with psychiatric illnesses.

Although medication is by no means the final and complete answer in the treatment of psychiatric disorders, it is an important component of treatment in many cases. The use of medications in psychiatry has contributed significantly to reducing the length of time that some people need to spend in the hospital and has allowed large numbers of patients to live happy and productive lives. Additionally, many medications have been shown to have value in preventing recurrences of certain psychiatric illnesses.

In addition to beneficial effects, all medications also have certain unwanted effects, or side effects, and the drugs used in treating psychiatric illness are no exception. The following discussions of the different classes of psychiatric medications identify individual compounds in these classes and describe their therapeutic effects and their most common side effects, as well. Of course, it is impossible to list every possible side effect of each of the medications discussed. The purpose here is to help patients better understand psychiatric disorders and psychiatric medications. This information may be expanded upon and further clarified by individual discussions between patients and their therapists.

ANTIANXIETY AGENTS

This class of drugs, also known as minor tranquilizers, includes chlordiazepoxide (Librium), diazepam (Valium), meprobamate (Equanil), and phenobarbital, as well as a number of less commonly used medications. These drugs have a fairly generalized calming effect on the brain, and, in small doses, relieve nervousness or anxiety by this action. In larger doses, they may produce drowsiness or sleep. Although they may have some calming influence on patients with depression or psychotic illnesses, they lack the specific actions on the brain that are necessary to treat these conditions effectively. These medications are particularly useful in preventing convulsions and in helping patients who are withdrawing from alcohol. Generally, the antianxiety agents are most effective when used only for brief periods of time or intermittently, on an as-needed basis. The major disadvantage of this group of medications is that, when taken in regular daily doses over periods of months, they can produce dependence and addiction.

The side effects most commonly experienced with the antianxiety agents include drowsiness, fatigue, and loss of coordination. Less frequently, they may produce confusion, constipation, depression, blurred or double vision, disturbances in speech, or disturbances in sexual function. Patients who have been taking antianxiety agents in relatively large doses over prolonged periods may experience convulsions should they suddenly discontinue these medications.

ANTIPSYCHOTICS

Unlike the antianxiety agents, the antipsychotics—or major tranquilizers—have rather specific effects on the brain. It is believed that it is this specificity of action which is responsible for their very dramatic beneficial effects in psychotic illnesses.

Psychosis, or psychotic illness, is best defined as a disorder in which a person's abilities to think, respond emotionally, remember, communicate, interpret reality, and behave appropriately are impaired to the extent that he or she has difficulty functioning and meeting the ordinary demands of life. People with disorders of this type often have poor impulse control and exhibit frequent fluctuations in mood. Because of their impaired ability to interpret reality, they often believe things to be true which are not true, or they may see things or hear sounds or voices which do not exist. Although the origins and causes of illnesses of this type are not fully understood, many theories have grown out of the extensive research, and there is considerable scientific evidence that the basic factors involved are biologic and chemical abnormalities in the brain.

Normal brain function depends in part upon the presence of a number of chemical substances (neurotransmitters) in the brain. If the quantities of these substances are too large or too small, or if the brain is too sensitive or not sensitive enough to the effects of these substances, the brain does not function normally. The evidence strongly suggests that in psychotic illnesses, either there may be too much of one of these substances (such as dopamine or norepinephrine), or the brain may be too sensitive to the action of a certain chemical substance. All of the antipsychotic drugs act to reduce the brain's sensitivity to one or more of these chemical substances and thereby produce their beneficial effects.

There are many very effective antipsychotic drugs available. The most commonly used include haloperidol (Haldol), trifluoperazine (Stelazine), fluphenazine (Prolixin), perphenazine (Trilafon), thiothixene (Navane), thioridazine (Mellaril), and chlorpromazine (Thorazine). These medications are all very effective in removing the previously described symptoms of psychosis. They are particularly effective in relieving agitation and anxiety, in clearing the thought processes, and in ending hallucinations. A variety of drugs of this type have been developed because some patients will respond better to one medication than to another. It is occasionally necessary to treat a patient with several different antipsychotic medications before discovering that medication which is most effective and easiest for that particular patient to take. Although the side effects of the various antipsychotics are fairly similar, each individual drug may produce any given side effect to a greater or lesser degree. Therefore, if a patient on antipsychotic medication experiences a particular side effect which is disturbing to him, it is often possible to change him to a different antipsychotic and to avoid that side effect.

Possible side effects of the antipsychotic drugs include drowsiness or sedation, dizziness, fainting, rapid pulse rate, dry mouth, constipation, and difficulty in urinating. These medications may also produce parkinsonian symptoms such as restlessness, stiffness of the neck or of other muscles, and tremors of the hands and fingers. In addition, people taking antipsychotic medications may be overly sensitive to sunlight, and it is generally advisable for a person taking one of these medications to apply a sunscreen, such as aminobenzoic acid (PreSun) or sulisobenzone (Uval), prior to prolonged exposure to bright sunlight. In men, these drugs may impair the ability to have an erection or to ejaculate semen. Women occasionally experience breast enlargement, secretion of milk from the breasts, and missed or irregular menstrual periods. Again, changing to a different medication will frequently reduce or avoid these unwanted effects.

The length of time a person need continue treatment with antipsychotic drugs varies. Some people experience acute psychotic episodes and may need treatment with medication for a period of only weeks or months. Other people have illnesses which tend to recur, and they may require drug treatment over a period of years. Over the course of prolonged treatment with these medications, the physician will generally reduce the dosage gradually so that the patient may be maintained on the minimum effective dosage. Patients should never reduce their dosage or discontinue their medication without first consulting their physician, as this may lead to a recurrence of the psychosis and to the need for rehospitalization or other intensive treatment.

Antiparkinsonian Medications

There are several medications—trihexyphenidyl (Artane), diphenhydramine (Benadryl), and benztropine (Cogentin)—which are effective in treating such antipsychotic-drug-induced parkinsonian symptoms as restlessness, stiffness of the neck and other muscles, and tremors of the hands and fingers. These medications are sometimes given along with the antipsychotic medications in order to prevent the development of these symptoms, but since many patients do not develop parkinsonian symptoms, many physicians prefer to prescribe antiparkinsonian medication only if the symptoms become troublesome. One particular reason for not using antiparkinsonian medications routinely in all patients receiving antipsychotics is that these medications often produce blurred vision, dry mouth, rapid pulse, constipation, and urinary difficulties. After two or three months of antipsychotic drug treatment, antiparkinsonian medications can usually be discontinued without recurrence of parkinsonian symptoms.

ANTIDEPRESSANTS

Depression is perhaps the most common condition for which people seek help from mental health professionals. Depression may occur under a variety of circumstances and may span a wide spectrum of moods: from feeling sad and "down," to feeling completely hopeless and helpless. Many depressions follow a disappointment in life, the loss of a job, or the death of a close friend or relative. Some depressions occur in response to a life crisis and pass spontaneously or with the help of psychotherapy. Most people experience mild forms of depression at different times in their lives. The more serious forms of depression, however, interfere with a person's ability to enjoy life, and are more prolonged. The latter are often accompanied by a number of symptoms in addition to feeling "down," including: fatigue, lack of energy, loss of interest, inability to enjoy life, persistent worry, anxiety, loss of appetite, loss of weight, difficulty getting to sleep, awakening during the night or too early in the morning, disturbances in sexual function, and physical symptoms in the absence of medical illness.

In addition to their wide ranges of severity and persistence, incidences of depression are further variable in that some occur for no obvious reason. That is, a person may become severely depressed without having previously experienced a loss or other life crisis; or he may tend to become depressed periodically—that is, every several months or several years. Also, while everyone's mood fluctuates in response to their life experiences, some people have a disorder of mood regulation wherein they may experience repeated "highs" (periods of mania) or "lows" (periods of depression), or alternate between the two ends of the mood spectrum. Certain of the mood-regulating disorders are classified as manic-depressive illness. During manic periods, people may experience confusion, racing thoughts, rapid speech, poor judgment, anxiety, strange thoughts, and auditory or visual hallucinations.

It is generally believed that people who suffer more severe forms of depression may have an abnormality in brain functioning or chemistry. This abnormality is generally felt to be related to a deficit of a certain chemical substance (such as norepinephrine) in the brain. Conversely, those people who have manic episodes may have an excessive amount of norepinephrine or dopamine in the brain. Not all depressive illnesses need to be treated with medication, but many respond best to treatment which combines medication and psychotherapy. The medications which are beneficial in the treatment of depression all act to increase the amount or effectiveness of certain catecholamines in the brain; those useful in treating mania curb the actions of these substances.

There are two major groups of effective antidepressant drugs, tricyclics and MAO inhibitors. The compounds in both groups bring about fairly similar beneficial effects, but the two groups differ in their side effects.

Tricyclic Antidepressants

The tricyclic antidepressants include the following commonly known medications: amitriptyline (Elavil), imipramine (Tofranil), doxepin (Sinequan), and desipramine (Norpramin). These are all quite effective and usually bring about their antidepressant effect within 2 to 4 weeks. However, it is generally necessary to take one of these medications for a period of 6 to 12 months, and should a person discontinue the medication too soon, the depression may recur. There are a fairly large number of drugs in this category because, again, therapeutic response to and side effects with the different tricyclics vary from one individual to another. Many people experience minor side effects when they first start treatment with one of these medications, and the side effects usually diminish or disappear as the person becomes accustomed to the drug. The tricyclics may produce the following side effects: drowsiness, excitement, anxiety, dry mouth, blurred vision, constipation, difficulty in urinating, dizziness, rapid pulse rate, and weight gain. Men occasionally experience difficulties with erection or ejaculation of semen while taking these medicines. Women occasionally have breast discharges or irregular or missed menstrual periods.

MAO Inhibitors

The monoamine oxidase, or MAO, inhibitors accomplish the same antidepressant effect as the tricyclics, but their chemical mechanism of action is somewhat different. Therefore, they may be useful in cases where the tricyclic antidepressants have not been effective. The two more commonly used MAO inhibitors are phenelzine (Nardil) and tranylcypromine (Parnate).

The major disadvantages of the MAO inhibitors are the dietary and medication restrictions they impose. Patients taking these antidepressants must not consume pickled herring, sardines, anchovies, chicken livers, canned or processed meats, pods of broad beans, canned figs, yeast extract, or fermented beverages such as wine or beer (although they may occasionally have a single cocktail or two or three ounces of white wine). While being treated with MAO inhibitors, one should not eat more than two ounces of sour cream, yogurt, cottage cheese, American cheese, or mild Swiss Cheese per day. All other cheeses, cheese products, or food products whose manufacturing process involves fermentation should be avoided in the diet. Patients on these medications should not eat more than two ounces of chocolate per day. They should also either drink decaffeinated coffee or limit their intake of regular coffee to two cups per day.

Prior to taking any medication for any intercurrent illness, a patient taking an MAO inhibitor antidepressant should first consult the physician who prescribed the antidepressant to determine whether it is safe to combine any other medication with it. If a person taking an MAO antidepressant develops a cold, the following medications may generally be safely used: aspirin, acetominophen (Tylenol), guaifenesin (Robitussin syrup), and cepylpyridinium (Cepacol gargle). Patients being treated with MAO antidepressants should not use nasal decongestants in the form of nose drops, cough syrups, or cold remedies. Diet pills and stimulant drugs of all types must also be avoided.

The abovementioned foods and various medications must be avoided while one is taking MAO inhibitors as these foods or medications may interact with the antidepressant to produce high blood pressure or a severe headache. A patient taking an MAO inhibitor who violates these dietary and medication restrictions may become severely ill and could possibly suffer brain damage. If one does follow these recommendations carefully, the MAO inhibitors are quite safe and effective, and their side effects are frequently far less troublesome than those of the tricyclic antidepressants. The following side effects may occur during treatment with an MAO inhibitor and are unrelated to dietary restrictions previously discussed: drowsiness, fatigue, dizziness, faintness, and dry mouth. Generally, MAO inhibitors and tricyclics should not be given simultaneously, and, except under special circumstances, a person should discontinue all medication for several days before changing from one type of anti-depressant to another.

MOOD-STABILIZING DRUG: LITHIUM CARBONATE

Lithium carbonate is a simple chemical compound known as a salt and is the least expensive of all medications used in psychiatry. It is often referred to simply as lithium (or by one of its trade names, such as Eskalith). People whose mood fluctuates widely, with recurrent "highs" and "lows," may benefit significantly from treatment with lithium. It is especially effective in preventing highs (manic episodes) and is also effective, in conjunction with other medications, in treating acute manic episodes. Lithium is frequently helpful in preventing recurrence of depression; it may also be useful as an adjunct to other medications in the treatment of certain depressive illnesses.

The quantity of lithium in the blood or saliva of patients is easily measured, and this measurement is a necessary part of treatment with this medication. It is generally agreed that the range of effective blood levels of lithium is 0.6 to 1.2 mEq/liter. Blood levels of lithium must be measured during the interval of from 10 to 12 hours after the last dose taken in order to avoid falsely high or falsely low results. Generally blood levels are measured once or twice weekly during the first month of treatment with lithium. After that, the blood level may be measured twice monthly for a month or two, and thereafter, once every one or two months. Before treatment with lithium is begun, certain medical examinations and laboratory tests are generally done to ascertain that the patient does not have any underlying medical condition which would make such treatment hazardous.

Unlike most other drugs used in psychiatry, lithium does not produce sedation or stimulation, and most people taking this medication over extended periods are not aware of any particular adverse effects or symptoms associated with its use. When first starting treatment with lithium, patients occasionally experience tremors of the hands or fingers, increased thirst, and increased urine production. Mild nausea, stomach upset, and changes in bowel habits may also occur. These symptoms can generally be avoided if the patient does not take lithium on an empty stomach, and it is therefore recommended that lithium be taken either at mealtime or with a snack. Adjustments in lithium dosage, or the temporary addition of another medication, will often end the tremors that some people experience.

More severe side effects with lithium generally indicate excessive dosage (too high a blood level) of the drug. These latter effects include: persistent diarrhea, vomiting, drowsiness, muscular weakness, and lack of coordination. If these symptoms appear, one should discontinue lithium treatment until he contacts his physician. A patient on lithium who develops the "flu" or any other physical illness accompanied by fever, loss of appetite, lowered fluid intake, or stomach upset should stop taking lithium and contact his physician.

CONCLUSION

Favorable response to psychiatric treatment requires active participation by the patient, both in psychotherapy and in properly taking medications which may be prescribed. The better informed the patient, the more able he is to follow the prescribed regimen and thereby benefit from treatment. The material presented in this chapter is offered as a guideline for the therapist in explaining to his or her patient the biologic bases of certain psychiatric illnesses and the rationale of pharmacotherapy in alleviating and facilitating recovery from a wide variety of emotional disorders.

REFERENCES

1. Blackwell, B.: Drug therapy: patient compliance. *N. Engl. J. Med.* 289:249-252, 1973.
2. Snyder, S.H., Banerjee, S.P., Yamamura, H.I. et al: Drugs, neurotransmitters, and schizophrenia. *Science* 184:1234-1253, 1974.